Gout Diet

Contains Gout Inflammation Arthritis Relief Smoothie Recipes 1 & 2

100 Smoothie Recipes

HR Research Alliance

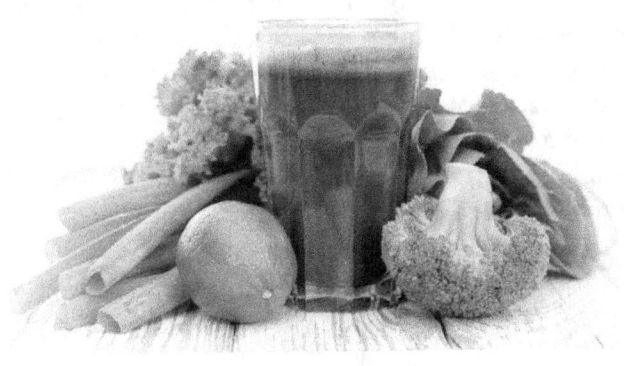

Table of Contents

You've Broc-To Be Kidding: Broccoli, Blueberry, Orange 39

Blackberry Cobbler: Blackberry, Almond 40

Lean, Mean, and Green: Spinach, Celery, Kiwi 41

P. B. & Green: Banana, Peanut butter, Spinach 42

Very Berry Cranberry: Raspberry, Cranberry 43

Feel the Beet: Banana & Beet 44

Super Booster Smoothie: Cranberry, Blueberry, Kale 45

Cauli-berry Smoothie: Strawberry, Cherry, Cauliflower 46

Pumpkin Pie Smoothie: Pumpkin, Banana, Cinnamon 47

Better Bloody Mary: Tomato, Strawberry, Basil 48

Papaya Creamsicle Smoothie: Papaya, Carrot, Banana 49

Avo-Cacao Smoothie: Avocado, Peanut Butter, Cacao 50

Green and Blue: Avocado, Blueberry, Spinach 51

A.K.C. Champion Smoothie: Avocado, Kiwi, Cucumber 52

Watermelon Sparkler: Watermelon, Cucumber, Lemon 53

Lemon Drop Smoothie: Lemon & Cucumber 54

Sweet Shirley Temple: Cherry, Orange, Ginger 55

P.B & K: Pineapple, Blueberry, Kale 56

Purple Power Punch: Red Cabbage, Cherry, Blackberry 57

Pina Caul-ada-flour Smoothie: Cauliflower, Pineapple, Orange 58

Hibiscus Citrus Quencher: Hibiscus Tea, Orange, Strawberry 59

Spiced Orange Smoothie: Orange, Turmeric, Cinnamon 60

Pineapple Zinger: Pineapple, Ginger 62

Maximum Mango Smoothie: Mango, Cayenne, Strawberry 63

Lettuce Be Cherry: Romaine Lettuce, Blueberry, Cherry 64

The Ultimate Cress: Watercress, Apple, Avocado 65

Dressed to Dill: Cucumber, Spinach, Dill 66

Black Forest Cake: Cherry, Banana, Almond 67

Spiced Carrot Cake: Carrot, Almond, Cinnamon 68

Energy Booster Cherry Smoothie 71

Healthy and Delicious Almond Cherry Smoothie 72

Banana Strawberry Smoothie 73

Creamy Green Avocado Cucumber Smoothie 74

Healthy Breakfast Fig Smoothie 75

Yummy Cantaloupe and Peach Smoothie 76

Green Kale and Kiwi Smoothie 77

Simple Creamy Mango Strawberry Smoothie 78

Tasty and Refreshing Pineapple Avocado Smoothie 79

Tropical Pineapple Orange Smoothie 80

Delicious Kale Banana Smoothie 81

Easy Watermelon Strawberry Smoothie 83

Energetic Lime Watermelon Smoothie 84

Zinger Papaya Ginger Smoothie 85

Introduction

Gout is a type of joint disease that is linked to the buildup of uric acid crystals in the fluids and tissues inside the body. It can be caused by the kidneys not being able to excrete uric acid from the body or from an overproduction of uric acid in the body. It is generally related to a poor diet, alcohol consumption, and the taking of certain medications, yet there are hereditary forms of the disease as well. There are about 3 million Americans who currently live with gout or gouty arthritis.

When a person suffers from acute gout, they may have a specific joint that becomes hot, swollen and red. The joint pain Is usually unilateral, meaning it doesn't affect the same joint on both sides of the body.

Most people with acute gout suffer from excruciating pain in the affected joint that can be easily managed by taking some type of NSAID drug (nonsteroidal anti-inflammatory drug) such as ibuprofen (marketed as Motrin or Advil) or naproxen sodium (marketed as Naprosyn or Aleve). Changes in diet and preventative medications can prevent an acute flare-up of gout but when a flare-up occurs, medications are generally necessary.

If acute gout is left untreated and the individual has repetitive instances of gout, this can cause a degenerative type of gout in the joints, which is also referred to as chronic gout or gouty arthritis. The goal of treatment in those suffering from gouty arthritis is to treat the pain of flare-ups and to keep the uric acid levels down as much as possible.

Symptoms of Gout As mentioned, just the presence of elevated uric acid levels doesn't mean you have gout and there are few symptoms. When gout has advanced to become symptomatic, the first symptom is usually the development of exquisite pain and swelling of the metatarsophalangeal joint of the great toe. It can come out of the blue or can follow an acute injury or an illness, such as a viral or bacterial infection. While gouty arthritis usually affects the metatarsophalangeal joint of the great toe, it can also present itself as pain and inflammation of the knee joint or an ankle joint. Attacks of gouty arthritis can affect the same joint the second time around or can skip to another joint in the body. If left untreated, the acute attack of gouty arthritis turns into a chronic case of gouty arthritis, which is more difficult to treat.

Usually only one joint is affected at any given time unless the disease is untreated and is really out of control. The time of onset to the time of resolution of symptoms is about 7 to 10 days. The pain goes from being excruciating to a dull, constant pain in the joint.

Tophi come from gout that has been allowed to be unchecked for many years. Tophi are deposits of uric acid that generally cluster around a joint. Tophi can disfigure the joint so that it is difficult to work with the affected area. Tophi may be debilitating but they are generally not painful.

Another complication of severe gout is the presence of kidney stones. Kidney stones occur when the uric acid is excreted in large amounts by the kidneys. If the urine is really concentrated, the uric acid precipitates out into a crystal that grows to become a painful renal stone.

While things like an elevated blood pressure, obesity, chronic renal disease, heart disease, and diabetes are not directly related to having gout, these symptoms and diseases are often seen together along with elevated uric acid levels. The typical gout patient is a male who is obese and who lives a sedentary lifestyle. His intake is likely to be high in red meat.

Causes of Gout

While the symptoms of gout appear to happen overnight, the ongoing process leading up to a painful attack of gouty arthritis comes on over a process of many months or years. The most basic cause of gout is an elevation of uric acid in the body (hyperuricemia). This is brought on by eating a diet high in purines (red meat is an example) or by failing to excrete uric acid to an adequate degree by the kidneys.

Uric acid is a breakdown product of purines. Purines are made by cells of the body and are taken in as part of the diet. Under normal conditions, the uric acid breakdown product is sent from the cells of the body to the kidneys, where it is excreted. The sufferer of gout tends to make more purines or eat more purines in the diet or fails to excrete it due to kidney disease.

The main causes of gout include the following:

• Eating high purine-containing foods

• Being obese

• Drinking too much alcohol, particularly beer

• Living a sedentary lifestyle

The following 50 recipes are taken from this book.

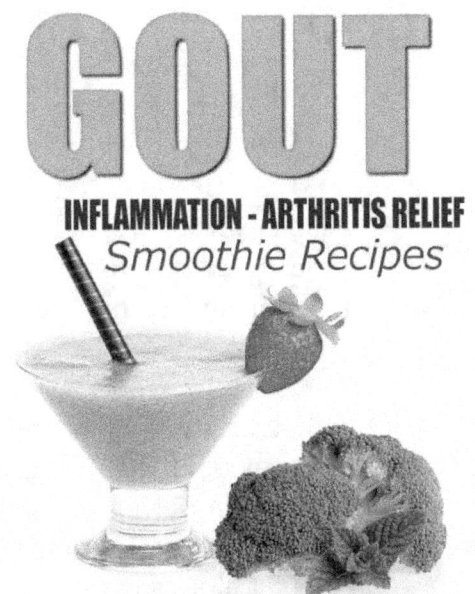

GOUT

INFLAMMATION - ARTHRITIS RELIEF

Smoothie Recipes

*50 Healthy Recipes That
Help Soothe Inflammation -
Anti Inflammation Recipes!*

HR Research Alliance

The Absolute Smoothie: Apple, Banana, Strawberry

Servings: 2
Ingredients
- 1 cup strawberries, halved
- 1 red apple, cored quartered, with skin
- ½ cup apple juice , unsweetened
- 1 banana, peeled
- 4-6 ice cubes

Directions
1. Combine ingredients in a blender. Cover and blend until smooth.

Nutritional Information (per serving)
- Calories 137
- Fat .5 g
- Carbohydrates 34.6 g
- Sugar 18.2 g
- Protein 1 g

Refreshing Classic: Oranges, Apple, Grape

Servings: 2

Ingredients

- 1 red apple, cored and quartered, with skin
- ½ cup apple juice , unsweetened
- 1 orange, peeled and separated
- 1 cup red grapes
- 4-6 ice cubes

Directions

1. Combine ingredients in a blender. Cover and blend until smooth.

Nutritional Information (per serving)

- Calories 303.9
- Fat .4 g
- Carbohydrates 77.9 g
- Sugar 51.4 g
- Protein 2.4 g

Banana Bahama Mama: Banana, Pineapple, Orange

Servings: 2
Ingredients
- 1 cup frozen pineapple chunks, unsweetened
- 1 orange, peeled and separated
- 1 banana, peeled
- ½ cup low-fat vanilla yogurt
- ½ cup coconut water
- 3-5 ice cubes

Directions
1. Combine ingredients in a blender. Cover and blend on high until smooth.

Nutritional Information (per serving)
- Calories 448
- Fat 0 g
- Carbohydrates 51 g
- Sugar 36 g
- Protein 6 g

Orange Power: Orange, Carrot, Turmeric

Servings: 2
Ingredients

- 1 orange, peeled and separated
- 1 ½ cup shredded carrots
- ½ tsp. ground turmeric
- ½ cup water*
- 4-6 ice cubes

Substitute with ½ cup apple juice, if desired.

Directions

1. Combine ingredients in a blender. Cover and blend until smooth.

Nutritional Information (per serving)

- Calories 142
- Fat 0 g
- Carbohydrates 35 g
- Sugar 22 g
- Protein 4 g

What a Plummy Pear: Plum, Pear, Blueberry

Servings: 2
Ingredients

- 1 pear, cored and chopped, with skin
- 2 plums, halved and pitted
- 1 cup frozen blueberries, unsweetened
- ½ cup low-fat blueberry yogurt
- ½ tsp. cinnamon

Directions

1. Combine ingredients in a blender. Cover and blend until smooth.

Nutritional Information (per serving)

- Calories 176.3
- Fat 1.6 g
- Carbohydrates 41.5 g
- Sugar 30.9 g
- Protein 2.6 g

Merry Berries and Plum: Cherry, Strawberry, Plum

Servings: 2

Ingredients

- 1 cup strawberries, halved
- 2 plums, pitted and halved
- 1 cup cherries, pitted
- 1 cup original almond milk, unsweetened
- 3-6 ice cubes

Directions

1. Combine ingredients in a blender. Cover and blend until smooth.

Nutritional Information (per serving)

- Calories 237
- Fat 3.4 g
- Carbohydrates 54.9 g
- Sugar 42.6 g
- Protein 4.4 g

Apple Pie: Apple, Cinnamon, Almond

Servings: 2
Ingredients

- 2 apples, cored and quartered, with skin
- 2 tbsp. creamy almond butter
- 1 cup original almond milk, unsweetened
- ½ cup low-fat plain yogurt
- ½ tsp. cinnamon
- ¼ tsp. nutmeg
- Pinch cloves
- Pinch of ginger

Directions

1. Combine ingredients in a blender. Cover and blend until smooth.

Nutritional Information (per serving)

- Calories 224.7
- Fat 10.6 g
- Carbohydrates 25.9 g
- Sugar 17.2 g
- Protein 10.1 g

Beet the Rush Smoothie: Beet, Strawberry, Raspberry

Servings: 2

Ingredients

- 1 small beetroot, trimmed and quartered
- 1 cup frozen strawberries, unsweetened
- 1 small banana, peeled
- ½ cup red raspberries
- ¾ cup orange juice

Directions

1. Preheat oven to 400° F.
2. While oven is preheating, wash and trim leaves off of beet. Cut into quarters and place on a baking sheet. Bake for 30 minutes, or until soft.
3. Combine ingredients in a blender. Cover and blend until smooth.

Nutritional Information (per serving)

- Calories 146.2
- Fat .8 g
- Carbohydrates 35.5 g
- Sugar 14.4 g
- Protein 2.5 g

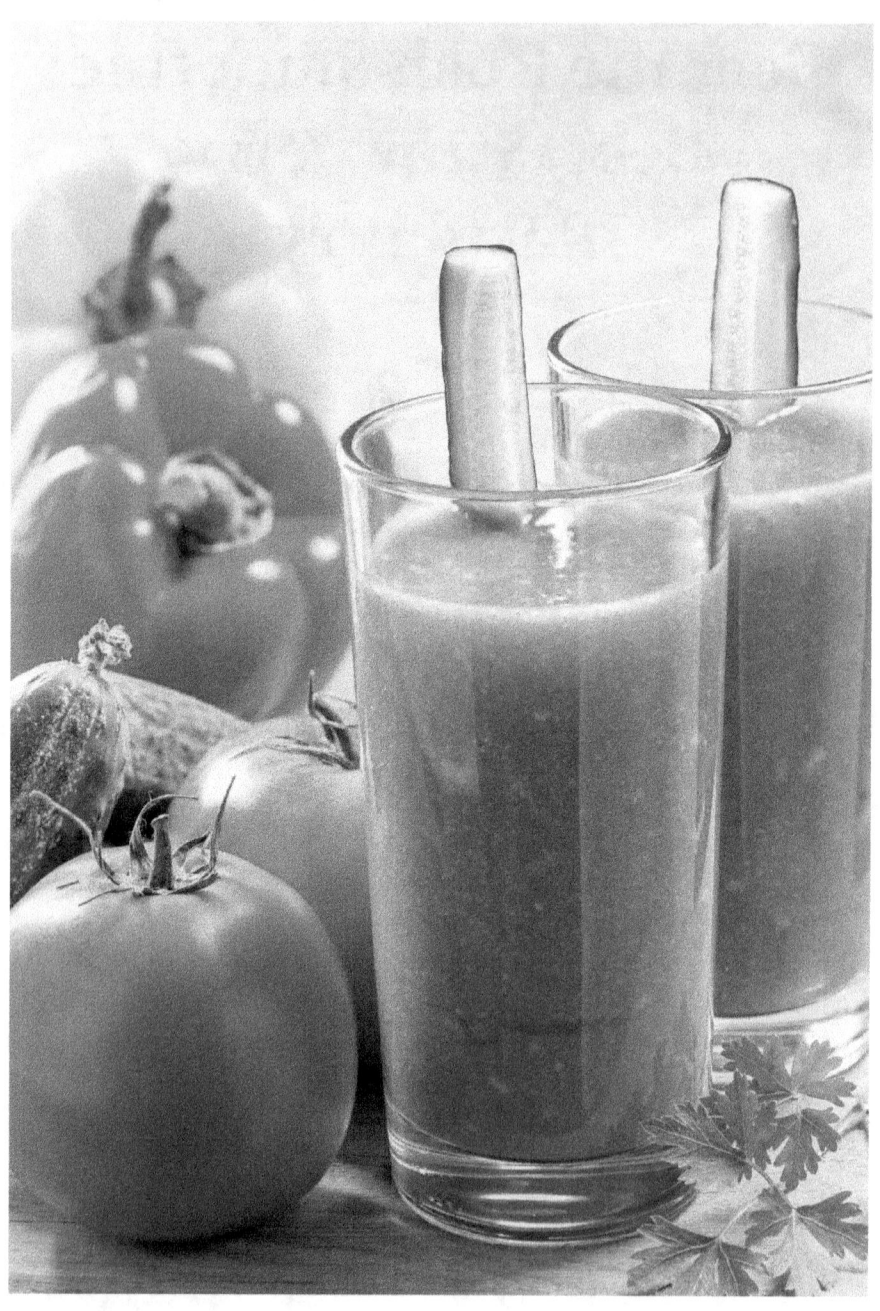

Watermelon-Basil Lemonade: Watermelon, Strawberry, Basil

Servings: 2

Ingredients

- 5 cups watermelon, cubed and seeded
- 1 cup frozen strawberries, unsweetened
- ½ cup cucumber slices
- ½ cup lemon juice
- 4 fresh basil leaves

Directions

1. Combine ingredients in a blender. Cover and blend until smooth.

Nutritional Information (per serving)

- Calories 164.2
- Fat 2 g
- Carbohydrates 39 g
- Sugar 28.4 g
- Protein 3.3 g

Creamy Cantaloupe: Cantaloupe, Pineapple, Banana

Servings: 2

Ingredients

- 1 cup cantaloupe chunks
- ½ cup frozen pineapple chunks, unsweetened
- ½ banana, peeled
- ¼ cup shredded carrots
- ½ cup coconut water

Directions

1. Combine ingredients in a blender. Cover and blend until smooth.

Nutritional Information (per serving)

- Calories 102
- Fat 0 g
- Carbohydrates 25 g
- Sugar 19 g
- Protein 2 g

Peary-Cherry: Pear, Cherry

Servings: 2
Ingredients

- 1 pear, cored and chopped, with skin
- 1 small apple, cored and quartered, with skin
- 1 cup frozen cherries, pitted
- ½ cup beet juice*
- ½ almond milk, original unsweetened
- 3-5 ice cubes

Substitute with cherry or apple juice , if desired.

Directions

1. Combine ingredients in a blender. Cover and blend until smooth.

Nutritional Information (per serving)

- Calories 135.3
- Fat .8 g
- Carbohydrates 33.1 g
- Sugar 21.4 g
- Protein 1.6 g

Peaches and Green: Peach & Avocado

Servings: 2
Ingredients

- 2 ripe peaches, pitted and quartered
- 1 ripe avocado, pitted and peeled
- 1 cup vanilla almond milk, unsweetened
- ½ small banana, peeled
- 1 tbsp. creamy cashew butter*

Substitute with almond or peanut butter, if desired.

Directions

1. Combine ingredients in a blender. Cover and blend until smooth.

Nutritional Information (per serving)

- Calories 250.2
- Fat 17.1 g
- Carbohydrates 26 g
- Sugar 12.3 g
- Protein 4.9 g

Sweet Potato Pie: Sweet potato & Banana

Servings: 2
Ingredients
- 1 medium sweet potato
- ½ banana, peeled
- 1 cup vanilla almond milk, unsweetened
- 2 tbsp. creamy cashew butter*
- ½ tsp. cinnamon
- Pinch of nutmeg
- Pinch of ginger
- Pinch of allspice
- 3-4 ice cubes

Substitute with peanut or almond butter, if desired.

Directions
1. Preheat oven to 350°F.
2. While oven is preheating, wash the potato. Pierce several times with a fork before baking it in the oven for 50 minutes, or until tender. Remove peel from potato and cool.
3. Once cooled, combine ingredients in a blender. Cover and blend until smooth.

Nutritional Information (per serving)
- Calories 179.8
- Fat 9.2 g
- Carbohydrates 21.7 g
- Sugar 6.2 g
- Protein 4.7 g

Sweet Peach Tea: Peach, Green Tea

Servings: 2
Ingredients
- 2 ripe peaches, pitted
- 1 cup water
- 1 green tea packet*
- 2 dates, pitted
- 1 small apple, cored and quartered, with skin
- 3-4 ice cubes

Substitute with peach tea, if desired.

Directions
1. Bring 1 cup water to boil, then let cool for approximately 2 minutes, or until 175°F. Steep one green tea packet in water for 1 minute. Remove packet and let cool.
2. Combine ingredients in a blender. Cover and blend until smooth.

Nutritional Information (per serving)
- Calories 139.7
- Fat .3 g
- Carbohydrates 36.2 g
- Sugar 29.1 g
- Protein 1.3 g

Sparkling Peach Spritzer: Peach, Grape

Servings: 2
Ingredients
- ½ cup apple juice
- 1 tbsp. lime juice
- 1 ripe peach, pitted and quartered
- 1 cup seedless green grapes
- 4-5 ice cubes

Directions
1. Combine ingredients in a blender. Cover and blend until smooth

Nutritional Information (per serving)
- Calories 107
- Fat .3 g
- Carbohydrates 27.8 g
- Sugar 16.3 g
- Protein 1 g

Cherry Citrus Smoothie: Pineapple, Cherry

Servings: 2
Ingredients

- 1 cup frozen pineapple chunks, unsweetened
- 1 cup cherries, pitted
- ½ cup orange juice
- ½ cup coconut water

Directions

1. Combine ingredients in a blender. Cover and blend until smooth.

Nutritional Information (per serving)

- Calories 157
- Fat 0 g
- Carbohydrates 37 g
- Sugar 29 g
- Protein 3 g

Sunrise Smoothie: Kiwi, Watermelon, Strawberry

Servings: 2
Ingredients
- 1 cup watermelon chunks, seedless
- 1 kiwi, peeled and sliced
- ½ cup strawberries, halved
- ½ cup original almond milk, unsweetened
- 4-5 ice cubes

Directions
1. Combine ingredients in a blender. Cover and blend until smooth.

Nutritional Information (per serving)
- Calories 64.8
- Fat 1 g
- Carbohydrates 14.6 g
- Sugar 6.7 g
- Protein 1.3 g

Better Birthday Cake: Vanilla, Spinach, Banana

Servings: 2
Ingredients
- ½ banana, peeled
- 1 banana, frozen
- 2 tbsp. creamy cashew butter*
- 1 cup vanilla almond milk, unsweetened
- ½ tsp. pure vanilla extract
- 2 cups spinach

Substitute with almond butter, if desired.

Directions
1. Combine ingredients in a blender. Cover and blend until smooth.

Nutritional Information (per serving)
- Calories 214.6
- Fat 9.4 g
- Carbohydrates 30.5 g
- Sugar 16.5 g
- Protein 5.1 g

Blue Raspberry Tea: Blueberry, Raspberry, White Tea

Servings: 2

Ingredients

- 1 cup low-fat blueberry yogurt
- 1 tsp. lemon juice
- 1 cup red raspberries
- 1 cup blueberries
- 1 cup water
- 1 white tea bag
- 3-4 ice cubes

Directions

1. Bring 1 cup water to boil, then let cool for approximately 2 minutes, or until 175°F. Steep one white tea packet in water for 1 minute. Remove packet and let cool.
2. Combine ingredients in a blender. Cover and blend until smooth

Nutritional Information (per serving)

- Calories 120.7
- Fat .3 g
- Carbohydrates 27.4 g
- Sugar 14.4 g
- Protein 4.2 g

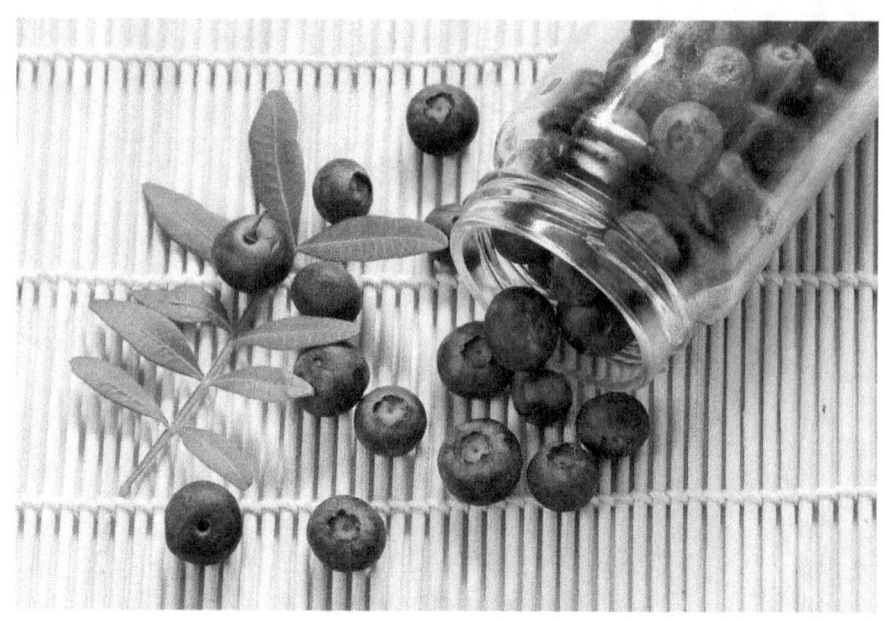

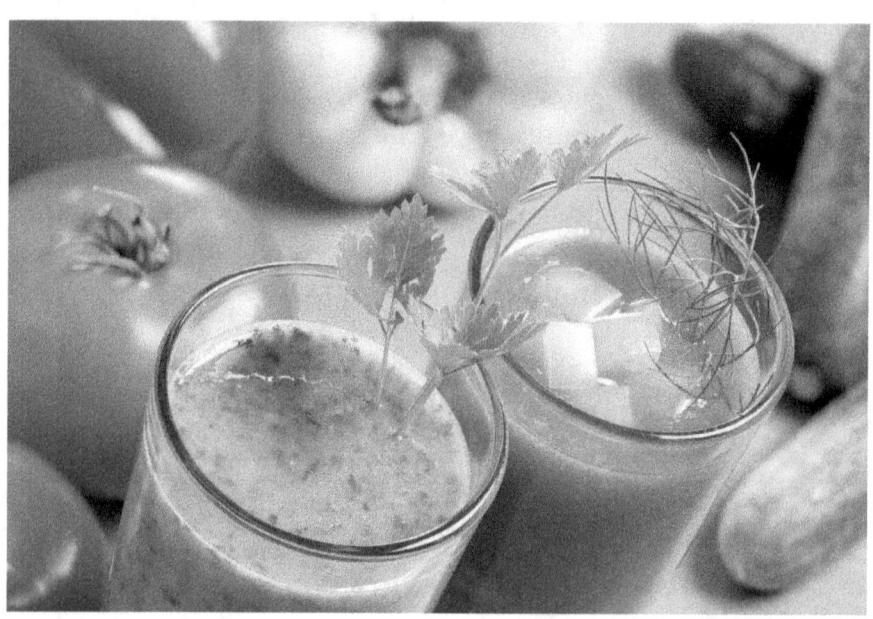

Blackberry Mango Tango: Blackberry, Mango, Honeydew

Servings: 2
Ingredients

- 1 cups frozen mango chunks
- 1 cup blackberries
- 1 cup honeydew melon chunks
- 1 cup coconut water
- 1 tsp. pure vanilla extract

Directions

1. Combine ingredients in a blender. Cover and blend until smooth.

Nutritional Information (per serving)

- Calories 108
- Fat 1 g
- Carbohydrates 25 g
- Sugar 16 g
- Protein 2 g

Mango Berry Smoothie: Mango, Blueberry

Servings: 2
Ingredients
- 1 cup blueberries
- 1 cup frozen mango chunks
- 1 cup original almond milk, unsweetened
- 1 tsp lemon juice
- 1 tbsp. raw coconut butter*
- 4-6 ice cubes

Substitute with almond butter, if desired.

Directions
1. Combine ingredients in a blender. Cover and blend until smooth.

Nutritional Information (per serving)
- Calories 155
- Fat 7 g
- Carbohydrates 24 g
- Sugar 17 g
- Protein 2 g

You've Broc-To Be Kidding: Broccoli, Blueberry, Orange

Servings: 2
Ingredients

- ¾ cup broccoli florets, de-stemmed
- 2 cups water
- 1 cup blueberries
- 1 orange, peeled and separated
- 1 cup orange juice
- 3-4 ice cubes

Directions

1. In a medium sauce pan, bring water to a boil. Boil broccoli for 7 minutes, or until tender. Remove from heat, drain, and let cool.
2. Combine ingredients in a blender. Cover and blend until smooth.

Nutritional Information (per serving)

- Calories 146.7
- Fat .6 g
- Carbohydrates 34.6 g
- Sugar 25.5 g
- Protein 3.5 g

Blackberry Cobbler: Blackberry, Almond

Servings: 2
Ingredients

- 1 ½ cups blackberries
- ½ cup original almond milk, unsweetened
- 2 tbsp. creamy almond butter
- ½ cup low-fat vanilla yogurt
- 1 tsp. cinnamon
- 1 tsp. vanilla extract
- 4-6 ice cubes
- Optional: add 1 Tbsp. raw honey for a sweeter smoothie

Directions

1. Combine ingredients in a blender. Cover and blend until smooth.

Nutritional Information (per serving)

- Calories 166.9
- Fat 9.1 g
- Carbohydrates 20.1 g
- Sugar 10.1 g
- Protein 4.3 g

Lean, Mean, and Green: Spinach, Celery, Kiwi

Servings: 2
Ingredients
- 2 cups spinach
- 2 celery stalks, chopped
- 1 kiwi, peeled
- 1 cup apple juice
- 4-6 ice cubes

Directions
1. Combine ingredients in a blender. Cover and blend until smooth.

Nutritional Information (per serving)
- Calories 96.5
- Fat .3 g
- Carbohydrates 22. 7g
- Sugar 14.1 g
- Protein 1.5 g

P. B. & Green: Banana, Peanut butter, Spinach

Servings: 2
Ingredients
- 1 large banana, peeled
- 2 tbsp. creamy peanut butter
- 2 cups spinach
- ½ low-fat yogurt, plain
- ½ cup original almond milk, unsweetened
- 4-6 ice cubes

Directions
1. Combine ingredients in a blender. Cover and blend until smooth.

Nutritional Information (per serving)
- Calories 172.3
- Fat 9 g
- Carbohydrates 21 g
- Sugar 10.3 g
- Protein 5.6 g

.

Very Berry Cranberry: Raspberry, Cranberry

Servings: 2

Ingredients

- 1 cup frozen cranberries
- ½ cup raspberries
- 1 small banana, peeled
- ½ cup original almond milk, unsweetened
- 2 tbsp. orange juice
- 4-6 ice cubes

Directions

1. Combine ingredients in a blender. Cover and blend until smooth.

Nutritional Information (per serving)

- Calories 127
- Fat 1 g
- Carbohydrates 28 g
- Sugar 15 g
- Protein 2 g

Feel the Beet: Banana & Beet

Servings: 2
Ingredients
- 1 medium banana, peeled
- 1 small beetroot
- 1 cup vanilla almond milk, unsweetened
- 1 tbsp. creamy peanut butter
- 3-4 ice cubes

Directions
1. Preheat oven to 400° F.
2. While oven is preheating, wash and trim leaves off of beet. Cut into quarters and place on a baking sheet. Bake for 30 minutes, or until soft.
3. Combine ingredients in a blender. Cover and blend until smooth.

Nutritional Information (per serving)
- Calories 132.8
- Fat 5.5 g
- Carbohydrates 19.4 g
- Sugar 10.8 g
- Protein 3.5 g

Super Booster Smoothie: Cranberry, Blueberry, Kale

Servings: 2
Ingredients

- 1 cup kale, raw and chopped
- 1 cup cranberry juice , unsweetened
- 1 cup frozen blueberries, unsweetened
- ½ banana, peeled
- 2 tbsp. orange juice

Directions

1. Combine ingredients in a blender. Cover and blend until smooth.

Nutritional Information (per serving)

- Calories 158.2
- Fat 1 g
- Carbohydrates 238 g
- Sugar 29.3 g
- Protein 2.3 g

Cauli-berry Smoothie: Strawberry, Cherry, Cauliflower

Servings: 2
Ingredients
- 1 cup cauliflower florets, de-stemmed
- 1 cup strawberries, halved
- 1 cup frozen cherries, pitted and unsweetened
- 1 small banana
- ½ cup low-fat plain yogurt
- 1 cup original almond milk, unsweetened

Directions
1. Combine ingredients in a blender. Cover and blend until smooth.

Nutritional Information (per serving)
- Calories 170
- Fat 1.8 g
- Carbohydrates 36.5 g
- Sugar 22.7 g
- Protein 6 g

Pumpkin Pie Smoothie: Pumpkin, Banana, Cinnamon

Servings: 2
Ingredients
- 1 cup pumpkin chunks*
- 1 banana
- 1 cup low-fat vanilla yogurt
- 1 tbsp. peanut butter
- 1 tsp. cinnamon
- Pinch of nutmeg
- Pinch of cloves
- 3-4 ice cubes
- Optional: tbsp. pure maple syrup
- Optional: ¼ cup pumpkin seeds

Substitute with 1 cup pumpkin puree, if desired

Directions
1. Preheat oven to 375°F. Bake pumpkin chunks for 50 minutes, or until soft. Peel and let cool.
2. Combine ingredients in a blender. Cover and blend until smooth.

Nutritional Information (per serving)
- Calories 212.1
- Fat 4.3 g
- Carbohydrates 33.6 g
- Sugar 21.7 g
- Protein 11.7 g

Better Bloody Mary: Tomato, Strawberry, Basil

Servings: 2

Ingredients

- 1 cup strawberries, halved
- 2 celery stalks, chopped
- ¾ cup tomato juice , unsalted
- ¼ cup water
- 3-4 basil leaves*
- 1 tsp. lemon juice
- 1/8 tsp. ground black pepper
- Pinch of cayenne pepper
- 4-6 ice cubes
- Optional: 2 celery sticks for garnish

Substitute 2 tbsp. dried basil, if desired

Directions

1. Combine ingredients in a blender. Cover and blend until smooth.
2. Optional: pour and garnish with celery sticks.

Nutritional Information (per serving)

- Calories 45
- Fat .4 g
- Carbohydrates 10.7 g
- Sugar 7.2 g
- Protein 1.5 g

Papaya Creamsicle Smoothie: Papaya, Carrot, Banana

Servings: 2

Ingredients

- 1 cup papaya, seeded and peeled
- 1 small banana, peeled
- ½ cup shredded carrots
- 1 cup coconut water
- 2 tbsp. orange juice
- 4-6 ice cubes
- Optional: 1-2 dates for a sweeter smoothie

Directions

1. Combine papaya and water; blend. Add banana, carrots, and ice. Cover and blend until smooth.

Nutritional Information (per serving)

- Calories 147.3
- Fat .5 g
- Carbohydrates 34.5 g
- Sugar 23.7 g
- Protein 2.3 g

Avo-Cacao Smoothie: Avocado, Peanut Butter, Cacao

Servings: 2

Ingredients

- 1 avocado, pitted and skinned
- 2 ½ tbsp. raw cacao powder
- 1 banana, peeled
- ½ cup low-fat vanilla yogurt
- 3 tbsp. creamy peanut butter
- ¼ cup vanilla almond milk, unsweetened
- 3-4 ice cubes

Directions

1. Combine ingredients in a blender. Cover and blend until smooth.

Nutritional Information (per serving)

- Calories 386.5
- Fat 24.5 g
- Carbohydrates 335.9 g
- Sugar 15 g
- Protein 12.5 g

Green and Blue: Avocado, Blueberry, Spinach

Servings: 2
Ingredients

- 1 ½ cup frozen blueberries, unsweetened
- 2 cups spinach
- 1 small avocado, pitted and peeled
- 1 cup original almond milk, unsweetened
- Pinch of cinnamon
- 3-6 ice cubes

Directions

1. Combine ingredients in a blender. Cover and blend until smooth.

Nutritional Information (per serving)

- Calories 206.2
- Fat 13.4 g
- Carbohydrates 23.7 g
- Sugar 9.9 g
- Protein 4.3 g

A.K.C. Champion Smoothie: Avocado, Kiwi, Cucumber

Servings: 2

Ingredients

- ½ avocado, pitted and peeled
- ½ cup apple juice
- 1 cup spinach
- 1 kiwi, peeled
- ½ cup cucumber slices
- 4-6 ice cubes

Directions

1. Combine ingredients in a blender. Cover and blend until smooth.

Nutritional Information (per serving)

- Calories 122.5
- Fat 5.9 g
- Carbohydrates 17.9 g
- Sugar 7.1 g
- Protein 2.2 g

Watermelon Sparkler: Watermelon, Cucumber, Lemon

Servings: 2
Ingredients
- 1 cup watermelon chunks, seedless
- ½ cup cucumber slices
- ½ cup green grapes
- 1 tbsp. lemon juice
- 2-3 mint leaves
- 4-6 ice cubes

Directions
1. Combine ingredients in a blender. Cover and blend until smooth.

Nutritional Information (per serving)
- Calories 57.5
- Fat .4 g
- Carbohydrates 14.3 g
- Sugar 11.1 g
- Protein 1 g

Lemon Drop Smoothie: Lemon & Cucumber

Servings: 2
Ingredients

- 1 cup low-fat vanilla yogurt
- ½ cup coconut milk, unsweetened
- ½ cup cucumber slices
- 2 tbsp. lemon juice
- 1 date, pitted*
- 4-6 ice cubes

Substitute 1 tbsp. raw honey, if desired.

Directions

1. Combine ingredients in a blender. Cover and blend until smooth.

Nutritional Information (per serving)

- Calories 102
- Fat 2.7 g
- Carbohydrates 15.8 g
- Sugar 10 g
- Protein 5.5 g

Sweet Shirley Temple: Cherry, Orange, Ginger

Servings: 2
Ingredients
- 1 cup cherries, pitted
- 1 cup orange juice
- 1 small banana
- 1 tbsp. fresh grated ginger*
- 4-6 ice cubes
- Optional: cherries for garnish

Substitute with 1 tbsp. candied ginger, if desired.

Directions
1. Combine ingredients in a blender. Cover and blend until smooth.
2. Optional: Pour and garnish with cherries on top.

Nutritional Information (per serving)
- Calories 149.3
- Fat .8 g
- Carbohydrates 36.5 g
- Sugar 20.3 g
- Protein 2.3 g

P.B & K: Pineapple, Blueberry, Kale

Servings: 2

Ingredients

- 1 cup kale, chopped
- 1 cup blueberries
- 1 cup frozen pineapple chunks, unsweetened
- 1 cup low-fat blueberry yogurt
- 4-6 ice cubes

Directions

1. Combine ingredients in a blender. Cover and blend until smooth.

Nutritional Information (per serving)

- Calories 211
- Fat 2 g
- Carbohydrates 45 g
- Sugar 32 g
- Protein 6 g

Purple Power Punch: Red Cabbage, Cherry, Blackberry

Servings: 2

Ingredients

- 1 cup frozen cherries, pitted
- 1 cup strawberries, halved
- ½ cup blackberries
- 1 cup red cabbage, chopped
- ½ cup juice orange juice
- 1 cup low-fat blueberry yogurt

Directions

1. Combine ingredients in a blender. Cover and blend until smooth.

Nutritional Information (per serving)

- Calories 247.7
- Fat 2.7 g
- Carbohydrates 53.5 g
- Sugar 41.7 g
- Protein 5.3 g

Pina Caul-ada-flour Smoothie: Cauliflower, Pineapple, Orange

Servings: 2
Ingredients

- ½ cup cauliflower florets, de-stemmed
- 1 ½ cup frozen pineapple chunks, unsweetened
- 1 cup coconut milk, unsweetened
- Optional: 2 pineapple wedges for garnish

Directions

1. Combine all ingredients in a blender. Cover and blend until smooth.
2. Optional: pour into glasses and garnish the rims with pineapple wedges.

Nutritional Information (per serving)

- Calories 89
- Fat 3 g
- Carbohydrates 17 g
- Sugar 11 g
- Protein 1 g

Hibiscus Citrus Quencher: Hibiscus Tea, Orange, Strawberry

Servings: 2

Ingredients

- 1 cup water
- 1 hibiscus tea bag
- 1 cup frozen strawberries, unsweetened
- 1 orange, peeled and separated
- 1 tsp. cinnamon
- Pinch of black pepper
- 4-6 ice cubes

Directions

1. Heat water to a boil then remove from heat. Steep hibiscus tea bag for 3-5 minutes. Remove bag and let cool.
2. Combine ingredients in a blender. Cover and blend until smooth.

Nutritional Information (per serving)

- Calories 56.8
- Fat .1 g
- Carbohydrates 14.5 g
- Sugar 9.6 g
- Protein .9 g

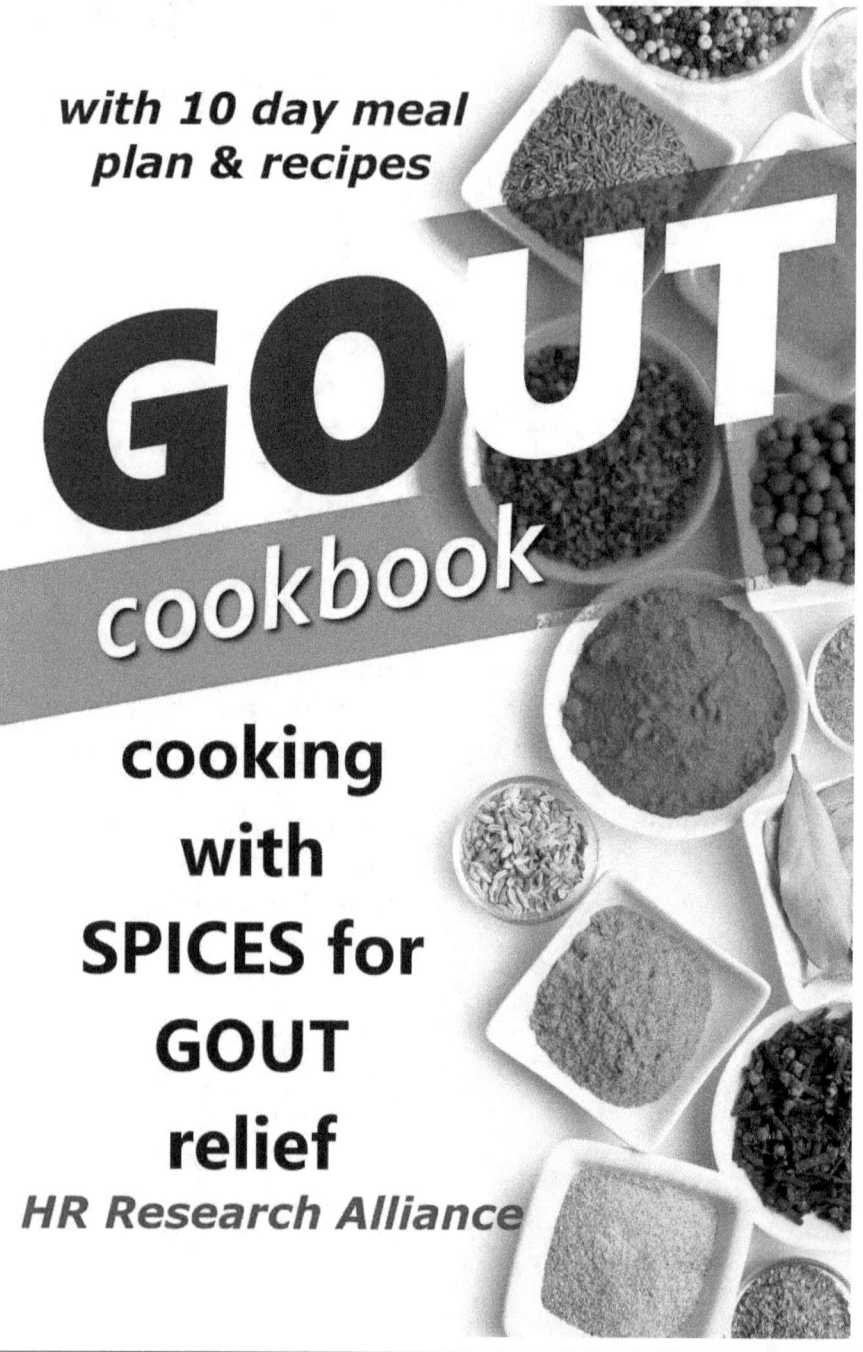

with 10 day meal plan & recipes

GOUT

cookbook

cooking

with

SPICES for

GOUT

relief

HR Research Alliance

Spiced Orange Smoothie: Orange, Turmeric, Cinnamon

Servings: 2

Ingredients

- 2 oranges, peeled and separated
- 1 cup cantaloupe chunks, peeled
- 1 cup original almond milk, unsweetened
- ½ tsp. turmeric powder
- ½ tsp. freshly grated ginger
- ½ tsp. cinnamon
- 4-6 ice cubes

Directions

1. Combine ingredients in a blender. Cover and blend until smooth.

Nutritional Information (per serving)

- Calories 103.6
- Fat 1.5 g
- Carbohydrates 16.4 g
- Sugar 18.7 g
- Protein 2.3 g

Pineapple Zinger: Pineapple, Ginger

Servings: 2
Ingredients
- 1 cup frozen pineapple, unsweetened
- 1 small banana, peeled
- 1 tbsp. freshly grated ginger
- ½ cup low-fat peach yogurt
- ½ cup coconut water
- Pinch of cinnamon

Directions
1. Combine ingredients in a blender. Cover and blend until smooth.

Nutritional Information (per serving)
- Calories 210
- Fat 7 g
- Carbohydrates 49 g
- Sugar 25 g
- Protein 2 g

Maximum Mango Smoothie: Mango, Cayenne, Strawberry

Servings: 2
Ingredients
- 1 cup mango chunks, peeled
- ½ cup frozen strawberries, unsweetened
- 1 banana, peeled
- ¼ tsp. cayenne pepper
- Pinch of cinnamon
- Dash of lime juice
- Optional: 1 tbsp. raw honey for additional sweetness

Directions
1. Combine ingredients in a blender. Cover and blend until smooth.

Nutritional Information (per serving)
- Calories 102.8
- Fat .4 g
- Carbohydrates 26.7 g
- Sugar 18.9 g
- Protein 1 g

Lettuce Be Cherry: Romaine Lettuce, Blueberry, Cherry

Servings: 2

Ingredients

- 1 cup romaine lettuce, chopped
- ½ cup cherries, pitted
- 1 cup blueberries
- 1 cup cherry juice
- 4-6 ice cubes

Directions

1. Combine ingredients in a blender. Cover and blend until smooth.

Nutritional Information (per serving)

- Calories 157.4
- Fat .1 g
- Carbohydrates 38.7 g
- Sugar 28.1 g
- Protein 2.3 g

The Ultimate Cress: Watercress, Apple, Avocado

Servings: 2
Ingredients

- ¼ cup watercress
- ½ small avocado, pitted and peeled
- 1 small banana, peeled
- 1 apple, cored and quartered, with skin
- 1 cup apple juice , unsweetened
- 3-6 ice cubes

Directions

1. Combine ingredients in a blender. Cover and blend until smooth.

Nutritional Information (per serving)

- Calories 185
- Fat 6 g
- Carbohydrates 34.9 g
- Sugar 10.5 g
- Protein 2 g

Dressed to Dill: Cucumber, Spinach, Dill

Servings: 2
Ingredients

- 2 cups cucumber slices
- ¼ cup lemon juice
- 5 sprigs of dill
- 1 cup spinach
- 1 cup low-fat plain yogurt
- 4-6 ice cubes

Directions

1. Combine ingredients in a blender. Cover and blend until smooth.

Nutritional Information (per serving)

- Calories 100.5
- Fat 2.2 g
- Carbohydrates 14 g
- Sugar 8.7 g
- Protein 7.7 g

Black Forest Cake: Cherry, Banana, Almond

Servings: 2
Ingredients
- ½ cup spinach
- 2 small bananas, peeled
- 2 tbsp. creamy almond butter
- 1/3 cup frozen cherries, pitted and unsweetened
- 1 cup vanilla almond milk, unsweetened
- 2 tbsp. raw cacao powder, extra for garnish
- 1 tsp. cinnamon
- 1 tsp. pure vanilla extract
- 3-5 ice cubes
- Optional: fresh cherries for garnish

Directions
1. Combine ingredients in a blender. Cover and blend until smooth.
2. Optional: pour into glasses and garnish with a light dusting of cacao powder and fresh cherries.

Nutritional Information (per serving)
- Calories 225.9
- Fat 11 g
- Carbohydrates 29.9 g
- Sugar 13.6 g
- Protein 5.5 g

Spiced Carrot Cake: Carrot, Almond, Cinnamon

Servings: 2

Ingredients

- 2 small bananas
- 1 cup shredded carrots
- 1 cup vanilla almond milk, unsweetened
- 2 tbsp. creamy almond butter
- ½ tsp cinnamon
- Pinch of powdered ginger
- Pinch of nutmeg
- Optional: 1 tbsp. raw honey for a sweeter smoothie
- 4-6 ice cubes

Directions

1. Combine ingredients in a blender. Cover and blend until smooth.

Nutritional Information (per serving)

- Calories 210.4
- Fat 10.5 g
- Carbohydrates 28.2 g
- Sugar 13.4 g
- Protein 4.4 g

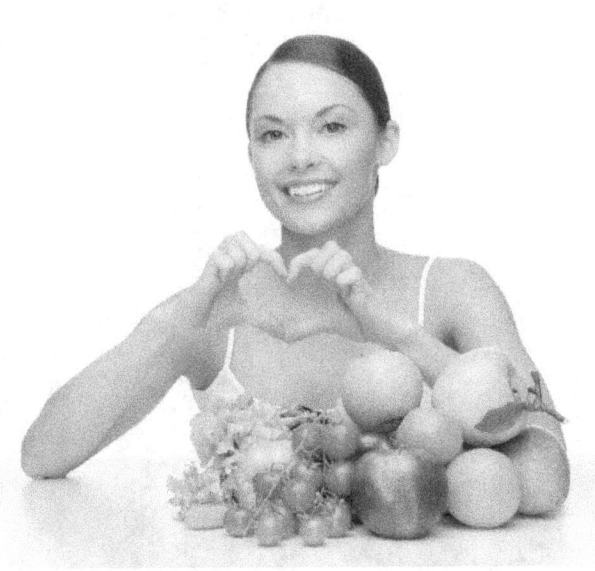

The next section is taken from this book.

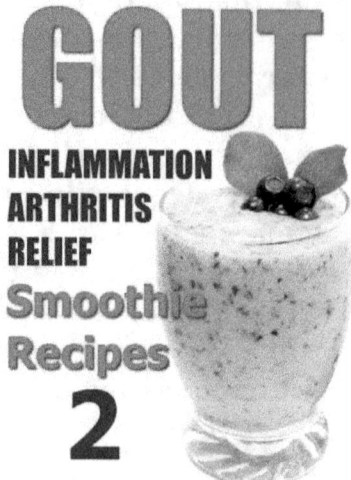

GOUT

**INFLAMMATION
ARTHRITIS
RELIEF**

**Smoothie
Recipes**

2

**50 Healthy Recipes That
Help Soothe Inflammation -
Anti Inflammation Recipes!**
HR Research Alliance

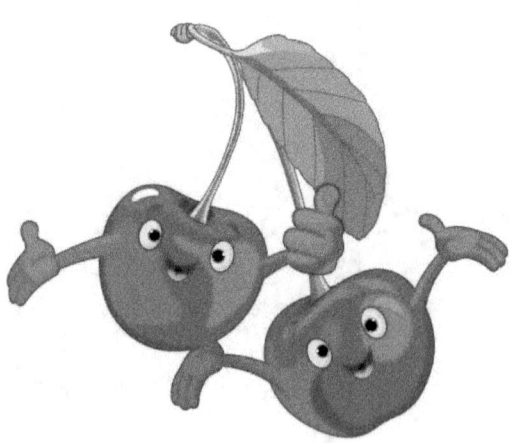

Energy Booster Cherry Smoothie

Total Time: 5 minutes

Serves: 3

Ingredients:

- 1 1/2 cup fresh cherries, pitted
- 2 dates, pitted
- 1 cup almond milk
- 1 banana

Directions:

1. Add all ingredients into the blender and blend until smooth.

Nutritional Value (Amount per Serving):

- Calories 235
- Fat 19.2 g
- Carbohydrates 17.6 g
- Sugar 11.0 g
- Protein 2.4 g
- Cholesterol 0 mg

Healthy and Delicious Almond Cherry Smoothie

Total Time: 5 minutes

Serves: 2

Ingredients:

- 2 tbsp ground flax seed
- 4 tbsp almonds
- 1/2 cup fresh cherries
- 1/2 cup ice cubes
- 1 cup almond milk, unsweetened

Directions:

1. Add all ingredients into the blender and blend until smooth.
2. Serve immediately and enjoy.

Nutritional Value (Amount per Serving):

- Calories 145
- Fat 0.9 g
- Carbohydrates 36.2 g
- Sugar 29.8 g
- Protein 2.0 g

Banana Strawberry Smoothie

Total Time: 5 minutes

Serves: 2

Ingredients:

- 2 ripe bananas
- 2 cups fresh strawberries
- 1 cup orange juice

Directions:

1. Add all ingredients into the blender and blend until smooth.

Nutritional Value (Amount per Serving):

- Calories 207
- Fat 1.1 g
- Carbohydrates 50.9 g
- Sugar 31.9 g
- Protein 3.1 g
- Cholesterol 0 mg

Creamy Green Avocado Cucumber Smoothie

Total Time: 5 minutes

Serves: 4

Ingredients:

- 1 avocado, remove seed and scoop out
- 1/2 cup filtered water
- 1 lime juice
- 4 tbsp cilantro
- 1 small cucumber, peel and remove seeds

Directions:

1. Add all ingredients into the blender and blend until smooth.

Nutritional Value (Amount per Serving):

- Calories 109
- Fat 9.8 g
- Carbohydrates 5.8 g
- Sugar 0.9 g
- Protein 1.2 g

Healthy Breakfast Fig Smoothie

Total Time: 5 minutes

Serves: 2

Ingredients:

- 4 fresh figs
- 1 tbsp flax seeds
- 1 medium banana
- 1 1/2 cup almond milk
- 5 tbsp oats
- 1 tsp cinnamon

Directions:

1. Add all ingredients into the blender and blend until smooth.

Nutritional Value (Amount per Serving):

- Calories 631
- Fat 45.4 g
- Carbohydrates 58.3 g
- Sugar 31.6 g
- Protein 8.4 g

Yummy Cantaloupe and Peach Smoothie

Total Time: 5 minutes

Serves: 4

Ingredients:

- 2 cups cantaloupe
- 1 cup ice
- 1/2 tbsp honey
- 10 oz light peach yogurt
- 1 cup orange juice
- 8 slices of peaches

Directions:

1. Add all ingredients into the blender and blend until smooth.

Nutritional Value (Amount per Serving):

- Calories 231
- Fat 1.9 g
- Carbohydrates 48.0 g
- Sugar 46.5 g
- Protein 7.9 g

Green Kale and Kiwi Smoothie

Total Time: 5 minutes

Serves: 2

Ingredients:

- 1 cup kale, washed
- 2 kiwi, peeled and sliced
- 1/2 cup ice cube
- 2 tbsp honey
- 1 cup milk
- 2 ripe bananas

Directions:

1. Add all ingredients into the blender and blend until smooth.

2. Serve immediately and enjoy.

Nutritional Value (Amount per Serving):

- Calories 293
- Fat 3.3 g
- Carbohydrates 64.9 g
- Sugar 44.0 g
- Protein 7.2 g Cholesterol 10 mg

Simple Creamy Mango Strawberry Smoothie

Total Time: 5 minutes

Serves: 3

Ingredients:

- 1 cup mango, diced
- 1 cup milk
- 1 cup strawberries
- 1 ripe banana

Directions:

1. Add all ingredients into the blender and blend until smooth and creamy.

Nutritional Value (Amount per Serving):

- Calories 158
- Fat 2.4 g
- Carbohydrates 33.3 g
- Sugar 26.2 g
- Protein 4.3 g
- Cholesterol 7 mg

Tasty and Refreshing Pineapple Avocado Smoothie

Total Time: 5 minutes

Serves: 4

Ingredients:

- 2 cups pineapple, cut into chunks
- 2 avocados, remove seed and scoop out
- 1 cup almond milk
- 1 large banana
- 2 cups chopped spinach
- 1 cup pineapple juice

Directions:

1. Add all ingredients into the blender and blend until smooth.

Nutritional Value (Amount per Serving):

- Calories 451
- Fat 34.2 g
- Carbohydrates 39.1 g
- Sugar 21.1 g
- Protein 4.8 g

Tropical Pineapple Orange Smoothie

Total Time: 5 minutes

Serves: 2

Ingredients:

- 1/2 cup pineapple chunks
- 4 tbsp coconut milk, unsweetened
- 3/4 cup fresh orange juice
- 6 tbsp vanilla yogurt
- 1/2 tbsp ground flax seed
- 1/2 banana

Directions:

1. Add all ingredients into the blender and blend until smooth.

Nutritional Value (Amount per Serving):

- Calories 200
- Fat 8.6 g
- Carbohydrates 27.2 g
- Sugar 19.7 g
- Protein 4.5 g
- Cholesterol 3 mg

Delicious Kale Banana Smoothie

Total Time: 5 minutes

Serves: 2

Ingredients:

- 2 cups kale, remove stems
- 1 banana
- 2 cups water
- 2 tbsp chia seeds
- 1/2 lime juice
- 2 cups pineapple chunks

Directions:

1. Add kale and water in blender and blend until smooth.
2. Now add remaining ingredients into the blender and blend again until smooth.
3. Serve immediately and enjoy.

Nutritional Value (Amount per Serving):

- Calories 168
- Fat 0.4 g
- Carbohydrates 42.1 g
- Sugar 23.5 g
- Protein 3.5 g
- Cholesterol 0 mg

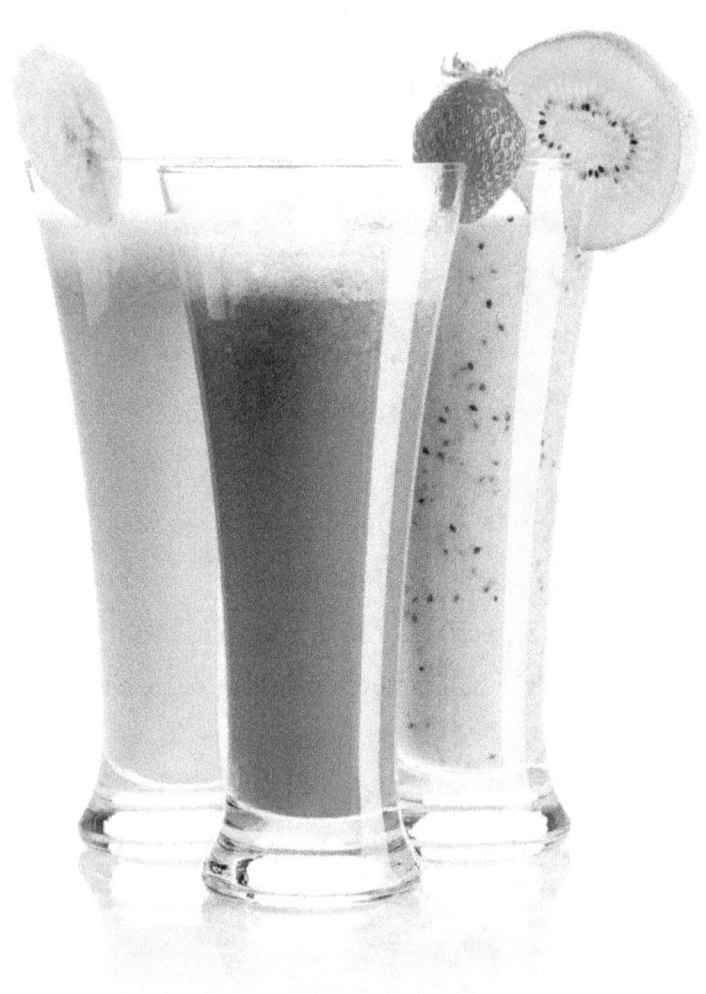

Easy Watermelon Strawberry Smoothie

Total Time: 5 minutes

Serves: 4

Ingredients:

- 4 cups watermelon chunks
- 2 cups strawberry
- 1 inch ginger
- 2 tbsp chia seeds
- 2 tbsp lime juice

Directions:

1. Add all ingredients into the blender and blend until smooth.

Nutritional Value (Amount per Serving):

- Calories 70
- Fat 0.5 g
- Carbohydrates 16.9 g
- Sugar 12.9 g
- Protein 1.4 g
- Cholesterol 0 mg

Energetic Lime Watermelon Smoothie

Total Time: 5 minutes

Serves: 2

Ingredients:

- 1 tbsp lime juice
- 2 cups watermelon chunks
- 3 fresh mint leaves
- 2 cups fresh strawberries

Directions:

1. Add all ingredients into the blender and blend until smooth.
2. Serve immediately and enjoy.

Nutritional Value (Amount per Serving):

- Calories 92
- Fat 0.6 g
- Carbohydrates 22.5 g
- Sugar 16.4 g
- Protein 1.9 g
- Cholesterol 0 mg

Zinger Papaya Ginger Smoothie

Total Time: 5 minutes

Serves: 4

Ingredients:

- 1 cup papaya chunks
- 1 inch ginger piece
- 3/4 cup milk
- 1 cup ice cube, crushed
- 1 cup pineapple chunks
- 1 tbsp lime juice
- 1 banana

Directions:

1. Add all ingredients into the blender and blend until smooth.
2. Serve immediately and enjoy.

Nutritional Value (Amount per Serving):

- Calories 85
- Fat 1.2 g
- Carbohydrates 18.3 g
- Sugar 12.5 g
- Protein 2.2 g
- Cholesterol 4 mg

Fresh Tropical Smoothie

Total Time: 5 minutes

Serves: 4

Ingredients:

- 1 cup papaya, cubed
- 4 cups almond milk
- 1 cup pineapple chunks
- 1/2 tbsp honey
- Ice

Directions:

1. Add all ingredients into the blender and blend until smooth.
2. Serve immediately and enjoy.

Nutritional Value (Amount per Serving):

- Calories 596
- Fat 57.4 g
- Carbohydrates 24.8 g
- Sugar 17.1 g
- Protein 5.9 g

Yummy Chocó Banana Smoothie

Total Time: 5 minutes

Serves: 4

Ingredients:

- 2 tsp cocoa powder
- 2 large bananas
- 1/2 cup ice cubes
- 2 tsp honey
- 1 1/2 cups milk

Directions:

1. Add all ingredients into the blender and blend until smooth and creamy.

Nutritional Value (Amount per Serving):

- Calories 119
- Fat 2.2 g
- Carbohydrates 23.4 g
- Sugar 15.3 g
- Protein 3.9 g
- Cholesterol 8 mg

Cool and Creamy Pumpkin Banana Smoothie

Total Time: 5 minutes

Serves: 2

Ingredients:

- 1 cup can pumpkin
- 1 banana
- Ground nutmeg
- 1 tsp pumpkin pie spice
- 6 ice cubes
- 1 cup almond milk
- 1 cup plain yogurt

Directions:

1. Add all ingredients except nutmeg into the blender and blend until smooth.
2. Garnish with ground nutmeg and serve.

Nutritional Value (Amount per Serving):

- Calories 460
- Fat 30.8 g
- Carbohydrates 39.2 g
- Sugar 24.0 g
- Protein 11.8 g
- Cholesterol 7 mg

Simple Mix Berry Smoothie

Total Time: 10 minutes

Serves: 2

Ingredients:

- 1 1/2 cup raspberries
- 3 kiwi, peeled and sliced
- 1 cup blueberries
- 2 cups orange juice
- 2 cups strawberries

Directions:

1. Add strawberries, blueberries and raspberries in blender and blend until smooth.

2. Then add orange juice and sliced kiwi and blend again until smooth.

3. Serve immediately and enjoy.

Nutritional Value (Amount per Serving):

- Calories 466
- Fat 1.6 g
- Carbohydrates 115.1 g
- Sugar 88.0 g
- Protein 4.9 g
- Cholesterol 0 mg

Healthy Immune Booster Smoothie

Total Time: 5 minutes

Serves: 2

Ingredients:

- 1/2 cup pineapple chunks
- 1 cup peaches
- 1 cup strawberries
- 1/2 cup plain yogurt
- 1 1/4 cups orange juice
- 6 ice cubes

Directions:

1. Add all ingredients into the blender and blend until smooth and creamy.

Nutritional Value (Amount per Serving):

- Calories 221
- Fat 1.3 g
- Carbohydrates 47.5 g
- Sugar 41.7 g
- Protein 5.5 g

Pink Grapefruit Raspberry Smoothie

Total Time: 5 minutes

Serves: 2

Ingredients:

- 2 grapefruit juice
- 2 cups fresh raspberries
- 2 fresh bananas

Directions:

1. Add all ingredients into the blender and blend until smooth.

Nutritional Value (Amount per Serving):

- Calories 210
- Fat 1.3 g
- Carbohydrates 52.0 g
- Sugar 28.8 g
- Protein 3.6 g
- Cholesterol 0 mg

Green Grape Avocado Smoothie

Total Time: 5 minutes

Serves: 2

Ingredients:

- 1/2 cup green grapes
- 1/2 avocado, remove seed and scoop out
- 1 banana
- 1 pear
- 2 tbsp chia seeds
- 2 cups water

Directions:

1. Add all ingredients into the blender and blend until smooth make sure chia seed nicely blend.

Nutritional Value (Amount per Serving):

- Calories 211
- Fat 10.2 g
- Carbohydrates 32.3 g
- Sugar 18.0 g
- Protein 2.0 g

Blueberry Chia Cherry Smoothie

Total Time: 5 minutes

Serves: 2

Ingredients:

- 1 cup fresh blueberries
- 4 tsp chia seeds
- 2 cups cherries, pitted
- 1 tbsp honey
- 2 cups coconut water

Directions:

1. Add all ingredients into the blender and blend until smooth.

Nutritional Value (Amount per Serving):

- Calories 145
- Fat 0.9 g
- Carbohydrates 36.2 g
- Sugar 29.8 g
- Protein 2.0 g
- Cholesterol 0 mg

Refreshing Apple Beet Smoothie

Total Time: 8 minutes

Serves: 4

Ingredients:

- 2 gala apple, diced
- 1 small beet, diced
- 1 cup filtered water
- 1 cup orange juice
- 12 ice cubes
- 1 1/2 cups fresh strawberries
- 3 tsp lemon juice
- 2 medium bananas

Directions:

1. Add all ingredients into the blender and blend until smooth.

Nutritional Value (Amount per Serving):

- Calories 145
- Fat 0.8 g
- Carbohydrates 34.7 g
- Sugar 24.1 g
- Protein 2.0 g
- Cholesterol 0 mg

Choco Cherry Smoothie

Total Time: 5 minutes

Serves: 2

Ingredients:

- 4 tbsp cocoa powder, unsweetened
- 2 cups cherries
- 2 cups almond milk, unsweetened
- 2 tbsp chia seeds
- 1/2 cup rolled oats
- 2 dates

Directions:

1. Add all ingredients into the blender and blend until smooth and creamy.

Nutritional Value (Amount per Serving):

- Calories 748
- Fat 60.7 g
- Carbohydrates 56.4 g
- Sugar 27.6 g
- Protein 11.8 g

Refreshing Melon Mint Smoothie

Total Time: 5 minutes

Serves: 2

Ingredients:

- 3 cups ripe honeydew melon
- 2 cup ice
- 20 mint leaves
- 5 tbsp lemon juice
- 1 tbsp honey
- 1 1/3 cup plain yogurt

Directions:

1. Add all ingredients into the blender and blend until smooth and creamy.
2. Serve and enjoy.

Nutritional Value (Amount per Serving):

- Calories 249
- Fat 2.7 g
- Carbohydrates 44.1 g
- Sugar 41.6 g
- Protein 11.0 g
- Cholesterol 10 mg

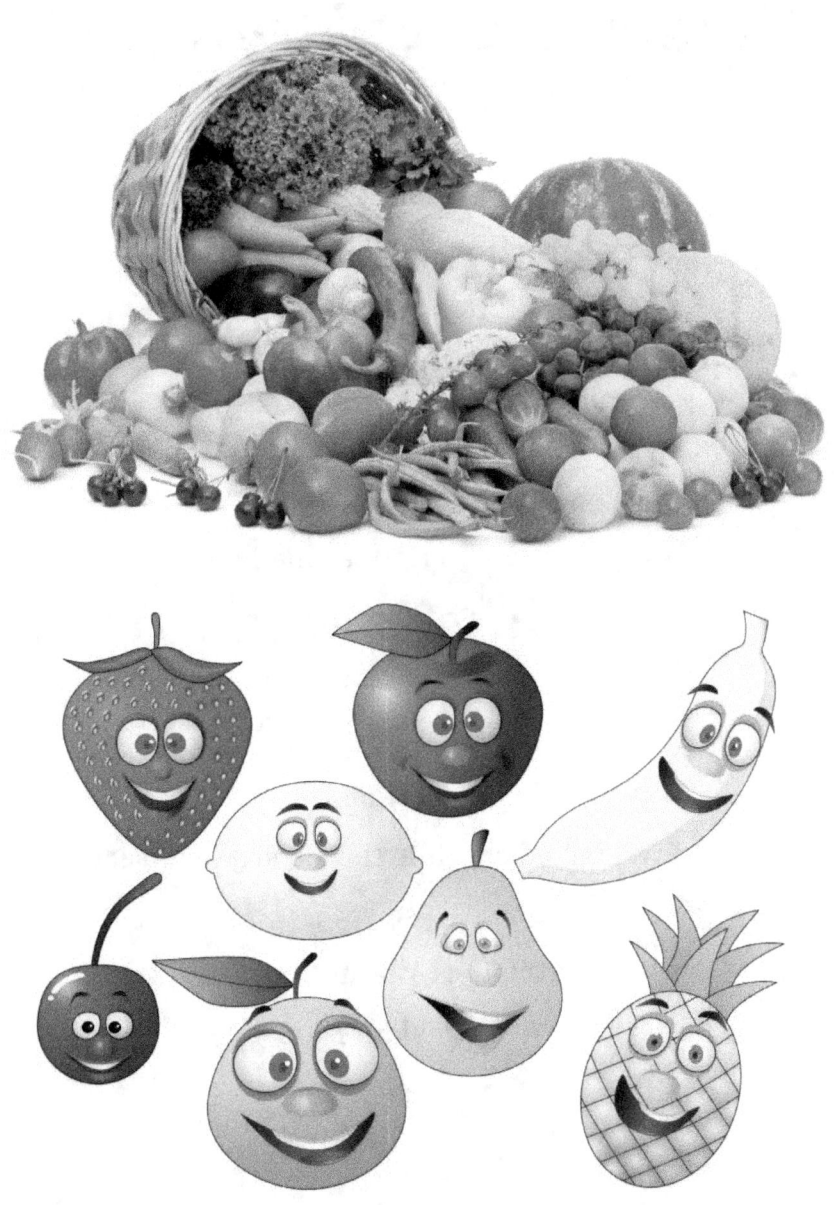

Zinger Ginger Honeydew Smoothie

Total Time: 5 minutes

Serves: 2

Ingredients:

- 1 cup honeydew melon
  - 1 inch ginger
  - 1 ripe banana
  - 1 cup watermelon
  - 1 cup cantaloupe
  - 1 cup almond milk

Directions:

1. Add all ingredients into the blender and blend until smooth.

Nutritional Value (Amount per Serving):

- Calories 408
- Fat 29.2 g
- Carbohydrates 39.9 g
- Sugar 28.9 g
- Protein 5.0 g

Exotic Guava Smoothie

Total Time: 5 minutes

Serves: 2

Ingredients:

- 1 guava, sliced
- 4 tbsp coconut milk
- 1 cup fresh raspberries
- 1 cup pomegranate seeds
- 1/4 cup ice cubes

Directions:

1. Add all ingredients into the blender and blend until smooth.
2. Serve immediately and enjoy.

Nutritional Value (Amount per Serving):

- Calories 132
- Fat 8.0 g
- Carbohydrates 15.4 g
- Sugar 7.7 g
- Protein 2.6 g

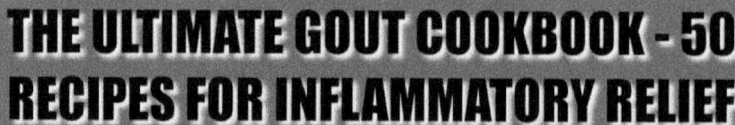

Vibrant Cranberry Banana Smoothie

Total Time: 5 minutes

Serves: 2

Ingredients:

- 1 cup cranberries
- 1 banana
- 1 orange
- 1 cup almond milk, unsweetened
- 6 ice cubes

Directions:

1. Add all ingredients into the blender and blend until smooth and creamy.

Nutritional Value (Amount per Serving):

- Calories 402
- Fat 28.9 g
- Carbohydrates 35.9 g
- Sugar 21.8 g
- Protein 4.2 g
- Cholesterol 0 mg

Apricot Mix Berries Smoothie

Total Time: 5 minutes

Serves: 2

Ingredients:

- 2 apricots, pitted
- 1 tbsp honey
- 1 cup almond milk
- 1 cup mix berries
- 1 cup ice cubes

Directions:

1. Add all ingredients into the blender and blend until smooth and creamy.
2. Serve immediately and enjoy.

Nutritional Value (Amount per Serving):

- Calories 365
- Fat 29.1 g
- Carbohydrates 27.6 g
- Sugar 20.8 g
- Protein 3.7 g

Easy and Tasty Pear Blueberry Smoothie

Total Time: 5 minutes

Serves: 4

Ingredients:

- 2 cups blueberries
- 1/2 cup water
- 1 pear, seeded and diced
- 1 tbsp honey
- 1 1/2 cup plain yogurt

Directions:

1. Add all ingredients into the blender and blend until smooth.

Nutritional Value (Amount per Serving):

- Calories 143
- Fat 1.4 g
- Carbohydrates 26.6 g
- Sugar 21.4 g
- Protein 5.9 g
- Cholesterol 6 mg

Healthy Celery Cucumber Smoothie

Total Time: 5 minutes

Serves: 2

Ingredients:

- 3 celery ribs
- 1 inch ginger
- 1 lemon juice
- 2 medium cucumbers

Directions:

1. Add all ingredients into the blender and blend until smooth.
2. Serve chilled and enjoy.

Nutritional Value (Amount per Serving):

- Calories 90
- Fat 0.7 g
- Carbohydrates 21.9 g
- Sugar 10.1 g
- Protein 3.9 g
- Cholesterol 0 mg

Carrot Celery Ginger Smoothie

Total Time: 5 minutes

Serves: 2

Ingredients:

- 2 medium carrots
- 4 celery sticks
- 1 inch ginger piece
- 1 lemon juice
- 3 green apples

Directions:

1. Add all ingredients into the blender and blend until smooth.
2. Serve immediately and enjoy.

Nutritional Value (Amount per Serving):

- Calories 199
- Fat 0.6 g
- Carbohydrates 52.2 g
- Sugar 37.8 g
- Protein 1.4 g

Fresh and Healthy Turmeric Pineapple Smoothie

Total Time: 5 minutes

Serves: 2

Ingredients:

- 1 inch fresh turmeric piece, peeled
- 1 cup pineapple, cut into pieces
- 1 tsp vanilla extract
- 1 cup almond milk
- 1 banana
- 1 inch fresh ginger piece, peeled

Directions:

1. Add banana, ginger, pineapple and turmeric in blender and blend until smooth.
2. Now add vanilla extract and almond milk and blend again until smooth and creamy.
3. Serve immediately and enjoy.

Nutritional Value (Amount per Serving):

- Calories 376
- Fat 28.9 g
- Carbohydrates 31.2 g
- Sugar 19.6 g
- Protein 3.8 g

Pain Relief Cucumber Pineapple Grapefruit Smoothie

Total Time: 5 minutes

Serves: 2

Ingredients:

- 1 cucumber
- 1 cup pineapple chunks
- 1 grapefruit
- 1 inch ginger piece

Directions:

1. Add all ingredients into the blender and blend until smooth.

Nutritional Value (Amount per Serving):

- Calories 84
- Fat 0.3 g
- Carbohydrates 21.5 g
- Sugar 15.1 g
- Protein 1.8 g
- Cholesterol 0 mg

Healthy Turmeric Pumpkin Smoothie

Total Time: 5 minutes

Serves: 2

Ingredients:

- 1 cup pumpkin
- 1 inch fresh turmeric piece
- 2 carrots, peeled
- 2 green apples
- 1/4 tsp cinnamon powder

Directions:

1. Add all ingredients into the blender and blend until smooth.

Nutritional Value (Amount per Serving):

- Calories 183
- Fat 0.7 g
- Carbohydrates 46.7 g
- Sugar 30.2 g
- Protein 2.5 g
- Cholesterol 0 mg

Anti Inflammatory Sweet Potato Ginger Smoothie

Total Time: 5 minutes

Serves: 2

Ingredients:

- 1 sweet potato
- 1 inch fresh ginger
- 2 carrots
- 1/2 cup pineapple chunks

Directions:

1. Add all ingredients into the blender and blend until smooth.

Nutritional Value (Amount per Serving):

- Calories 97
- Fat 0.3 g
- Carbohydrates 23.2 g
- Sugar 10.8 g
- Protein 1.9 g
- Cholesterol 0 mg

Fennel Cucumber Ginger Smoothie

Total Time: 5 minutes

Serves: 2

Ingredients:

- 1/2 fennel
- 1 large cucumber
- 1 inch fresh ginger
- 1/4 lemon juice
- 2 green apples
- 4 celery ribs

Directions:

1. Add all ingredients into the blender and blend until smooth.

Nutritional Value (Amount per Serving):

- Calories 139
- Fat 0.6 g
- Carbohydrates 36.3 g
- Sugar 25.7 g
- Protein 1.6 g

Everything You Must Know About Gout

HR Research Alliance

Gout

The Ultimate Guide

Simple Apple Peanut Butter Smoothie

Total Time: 5 minutes

Serves: 4

Ingredients:

- 2 medium apples, diced
- 2 tbsp peanut butter
- 2 cups ice cubes
- 1 tsp cinnamon

Directions:

1. Add apple, peanut butter and ice cubes into the blender and blend until smooth and creamy.
2. Pour into the glasses and sprinkle with cinnamon on top.

Nutritional Value (Amount per Serving):

- Calories 106
- Fat 4.2 g
- Carbohydrates 17.4 g
- Sugar 12.4 g
- Protein 2.3 g

Creamy Chocolate Avocado Smoothie

Total Time: 5 minutes

Serves: 2

Ingredients:

- 1/2 avocado, remove seed and scoop out
- 2 tbsp cocoa powder
- 1/2 tbsp honey
- 1 1/2 cups almond milk, unsweetened
- 3 tbsp peanut butter
- 1 medium ripe banana

Directions:

1. Add all ingredients into the blender and blend until smooth and creamy.

Nutritional Value (Amount per Serving):

- Calories 738
- Fat 65.7 g
- Carbohydrates 39.8 g
- Sugar 20.1 g
- Protein 12.7 g

Yummy Creamy Mango Avocado Smoothie

Total Time: 5 minutes

Serves: 4

Ingredients:

- 2 cups mango
- 1 avocado, remove seed and scoop out
- 1 tbsp honey
- 2 cups almond milk
- 1 cup plain yogurt

Directions:

1. Add all ingredients into the blender and blend until smooth and creamy.

Nutritional Value (Amount per Serving):

- Calories 539
- Fat 39.8 g
- Carbohydrates 44.6 g
- Sugar 35.9 g
- Protein 8.6 g
- Cholesterol 4 mg

Kiwi Coconut Smoothie

Total Time: 5 minutes

Serves: 1

Ingredients:

- 1 medium kiwi, peeled
- 1/2 banana
- 1/2 tbsp honey
- 1 can coconut milk

Directions:

1. Add all ingredients into the blender and blend until smooth.

Nutritional Value (Amount per Serving):

- Calories 131
- Fat 0.6 g
- Carbohydrates 33.3 g
- Sugar 22.7 g
- Protein 1.5 g
- Cholesterol 0 mg

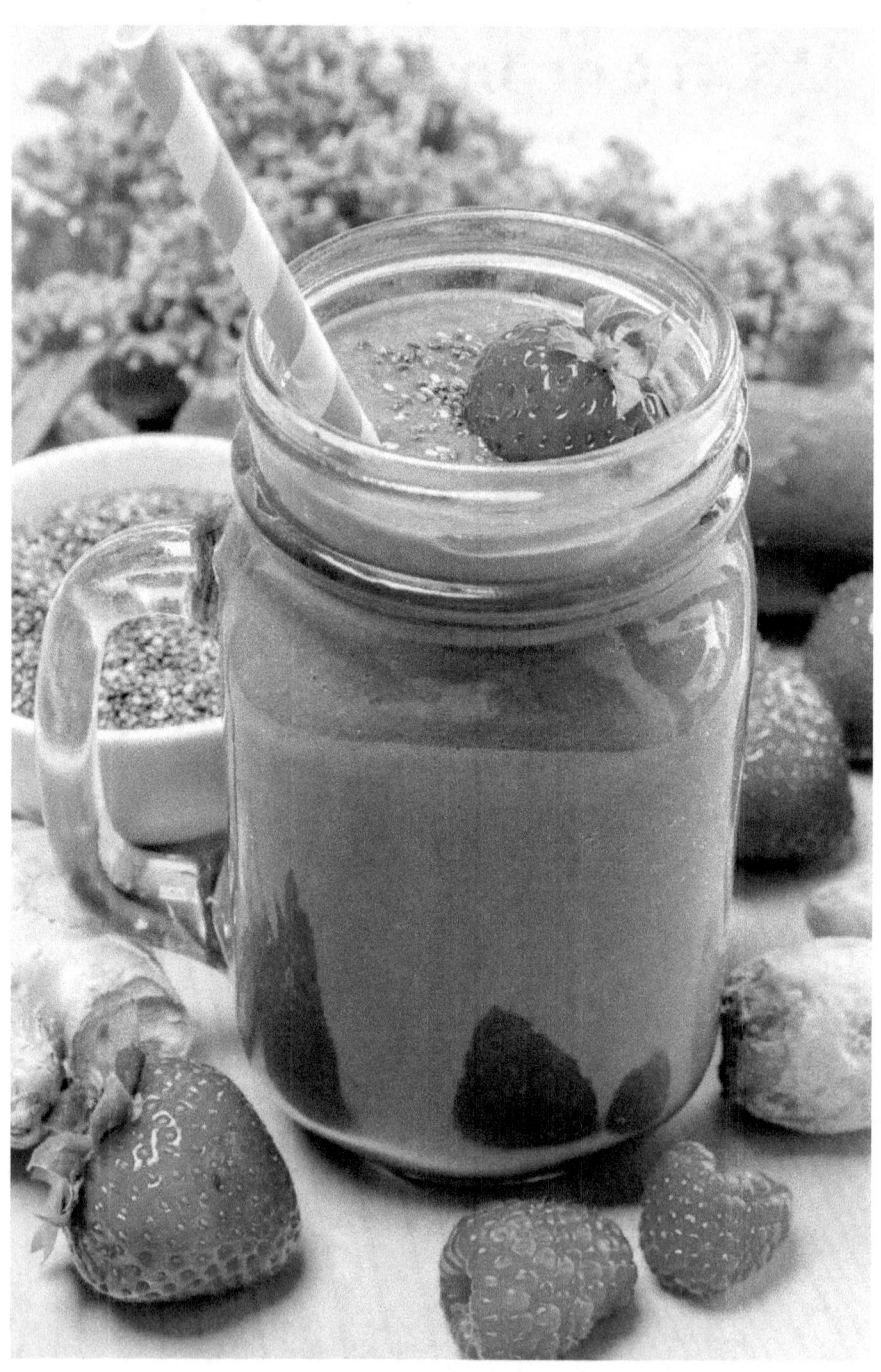

Breakfast Lime Spinach Smoothie

Total Time: 5 minutes

Serves: 2

Ingredients:

- 1 lime juice
- 2 cups spinach
- 1 tbsp hemp seeds
- 1 cup coconut water
- 1/2 cup strawberries
- 1 banana

Directions:

1. Add lime juice, spinach, coconut water, strawberries and banana into the blender and blend until smooth.
2. Pour into the glasses and top with hemp seed.
3. Serve immediately and enjoy.

Nutritional Value (Amount per Serving):

- Calories 71
- Fat 0.4 g
- Carbohydrates 17.3 g
- Sugar 9.1 g
- Protein 1.7 g
- Cholesterol 0 mg

Summer Refreshing Lime Honeydew Smoothie

Total Time: 5 minutes

Serves: 2

Ingredients:

- 2 tbsp lime juice
- 2 1/2 cup honeydew
- 1 tsp honey
- 1 cup coconut water

Directions:

1. Add all ingredients into the blender and blend until smooth.

Nutritional Value (Amount per Serving):

- Calories 87
- Fat 0.3 g
- Carbohydrates 22.2 g
- Sugar 20.1 g
- Protein 1.2 g
- Cholesterol 0 mg

Creamy Raspberry Chocolate Smoothie

Total Time: 5 minutes

Serves: 4

Ingredients:

- 2 cups raspberries
- 1 1/2 cup chocolate milk
- 1 cup ice cubes
- 1 tsp vanilla extract
- 2 tbsp cocoa powder, unsweetened
- 1 1/2 cups plain yogurt

Directions:

1. Add all ingredients into the blender and blend until smooth and creamy.

Nutritional Value (Amount per Serving):

- Calories 184
- Fat 5.1 g
- Carbohydrates 25.1 g
- Sugar 18.3 g
- Protein 9.4 g
- Cholesterol 17 mg

Yummy Orange Peach Raspberry Smoothie

Total Time: 5 minutes

Serves: 4

Ingredients:

- 2 cups fresh orange juice
- 2 peach, peeled and sliced
- 2 cups almond milk
- 1 1/2 cups raspberries

Directions:

1. Add all ingredients into the blender and blend until smooth.

Nutritional Value (Amount per Serving):

- Calories 385
- Fat 29.4 g
- Carbohydrates 32.1 g
- Sugar 23.4 g
- Protein 4.8 g
- Cholesterol 0 mg

Daily Refreshing Orange Strawberry Smoothie

Total Time: 5 minutes

Serves: 4

Ingredients:

- 3/4 cup fresh orange juice
- 2 cups strawberries
- 10 ice cubes
- 2 bananas
- 1 cup plain yogurt

Directions:

1. Add all ingredients into the blender and blend until smooth.

Nutritional Value (Amount per Serving):

- Calories 140
- Fat 1.2 g
- Carbohydrates 28.2 g
- Sugar 19.0 g
- Protein 4.9 g
- Cholesterol 4 mg

Healthy Romaine Lettuce Smoothie

Total Time: 5 minutes

Serves: 4

Ingredients:

- 4 cups romaine lettuce
- 2 cups plain yogurt
- 25 almonds
- 2 celery stalk
- 2 apples
- 2 bananas

Directions:

1. Add all ingredients into the blender and blend until smooth and creamy.

Nutritional Value (Amount per Serving):

- Calories 250
- Fat 5.8 g
- Carbohydrates 41.0 g
- Sugar 28.4 g
- Protein 9.8 g
- Cholesterol 7 mg

Green Broccoli Banana Lemon Smoothie

Total Time: 5 minutes

Serves: 2

Ingredients:

- 1 banana
- 1/2 tsp vanilla extract
- 1 tsp honey
- 1/2 lemon juice
- 1/2 cup almond milk
- 1/3 cup pineapple chunks
- 1 apple
- 1 cup broccoli florets

Directions:

1. Add all ingredients into the blender and blend until smooth.

Nutritional Value (Amount per Serving):

- Calories 291
- Fat 14.9 g
- Carbohydrates 41.8 g
- Sugar 27.3 g
- Protein 3.7 g
- Cholesterol 0 mg

Frosty Peach Grape Smoothie

Total Time: 5 minutes

Serves: 4

Ingredients:

- 1 1/2 cups baby spinach
- 2 cups coconut water
- 1 cup plain yogurt
- 1/2 ripe banana
- 1 cup grapes
- 1 1/2 cups peaches

Directions:

1. Add all ingredients into the blender and blend until smooth and creamy.

Nutritional Value (Amount per Serving):

- Calories 97
- Fat 1.1 g
- Carbohydrates 17.3 g
- Sugar 15.1 g
- Protein 4.6 g
- Cholesterol 4 mg

Zinger Ginger Pear Smoothie

Total Time: 5 minutes

Serves: 4

Ingredients:

- 1 tsp fresh ginger, grated
  - 2 cups pears
  - 1 tsp vanilla extract
  - 1 tsp honey
  - 2 tbsp almond butter
  - 1 cup plain yogurt
  - 2 cups spinach
- 2 cups almond milk, unsweetened

Directions:

1. Add all ingredients into the blender and blend until smooth.

Nutritional Value (Amount per Serving):

- Calories 428
- Fat 34.1 g
- Carbohydrates 27.1 g
- Sugar 18.2 g
- Protein 8.7 g
- Cholesterol 4 mg

Your Reviews are greatly appreciated, and your experiences help others cope with their own. Please do share, and help others by leaving your experiences with gout, in the review section of this book.

More educational, & diet books on gout & inflammation that you may find helpful.

Research these, and other related titles on Amazon.

Gout Treatment

Gout Diet

GOUT

Prevention

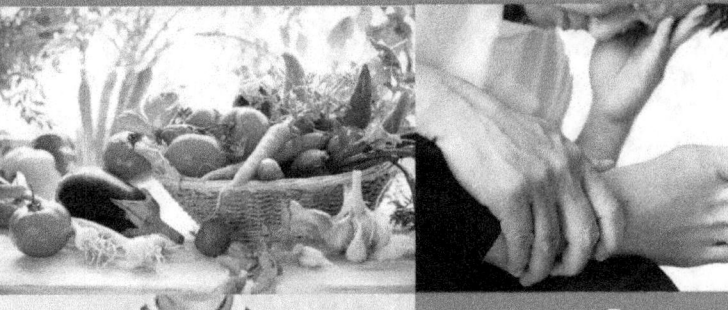

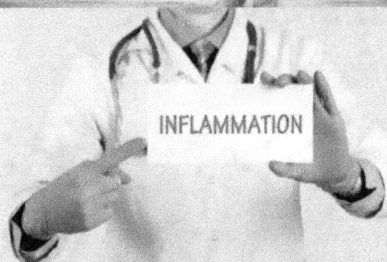

INFLAMMATION

JT Thorpe

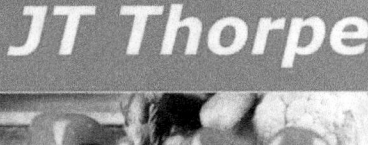

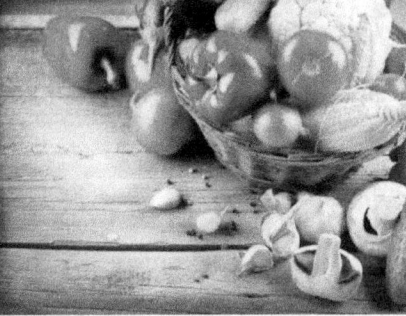

Gout Relief

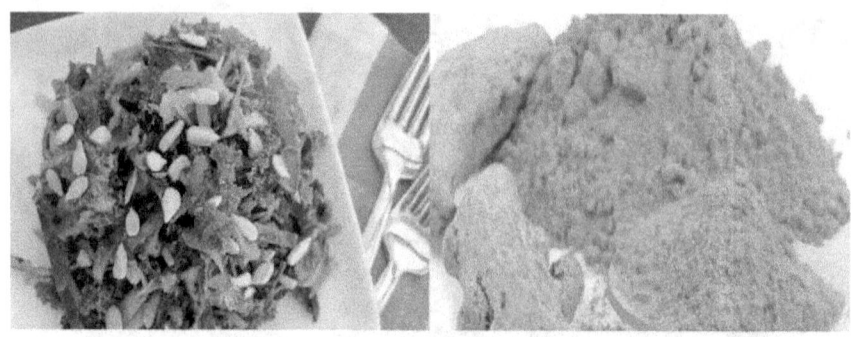

ANTI - INFLAMMATORY

COOKBOOK

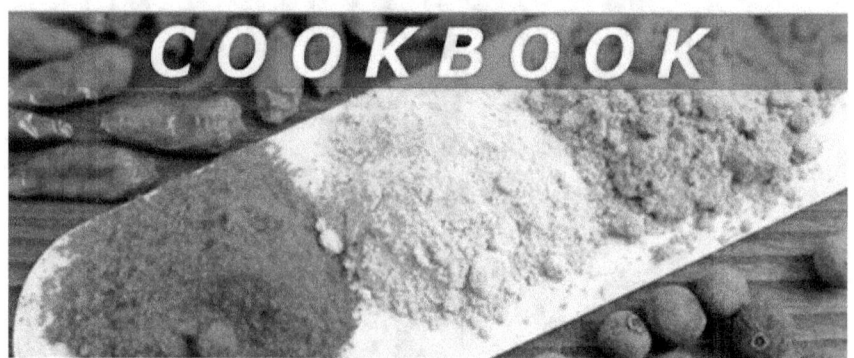

50

Slow Cooker Recipes With Anti - Inflammatory Ingredients

GREAT FOR GOUT RELIEF!

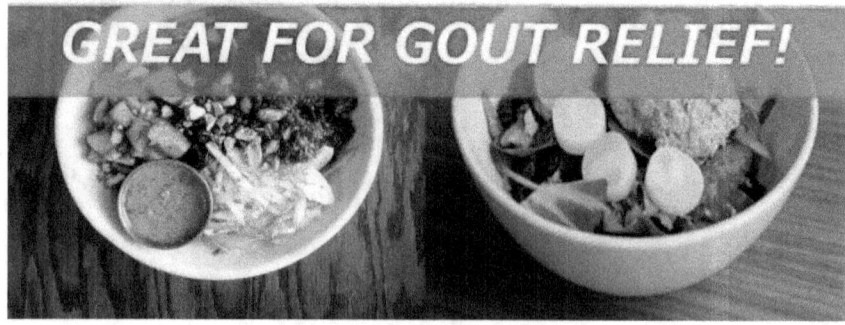

ANTI
INFLAMMATION
GUIDE

HR Research Alliance

INFLAMMATION

The 30 Day Elimination Inflammation Protocol

Anti Inflammatory Foods - Lifestyle Changes - Tips - Anti Inflammation Cooking - Daily - Weekly - Meal Plans - & More...

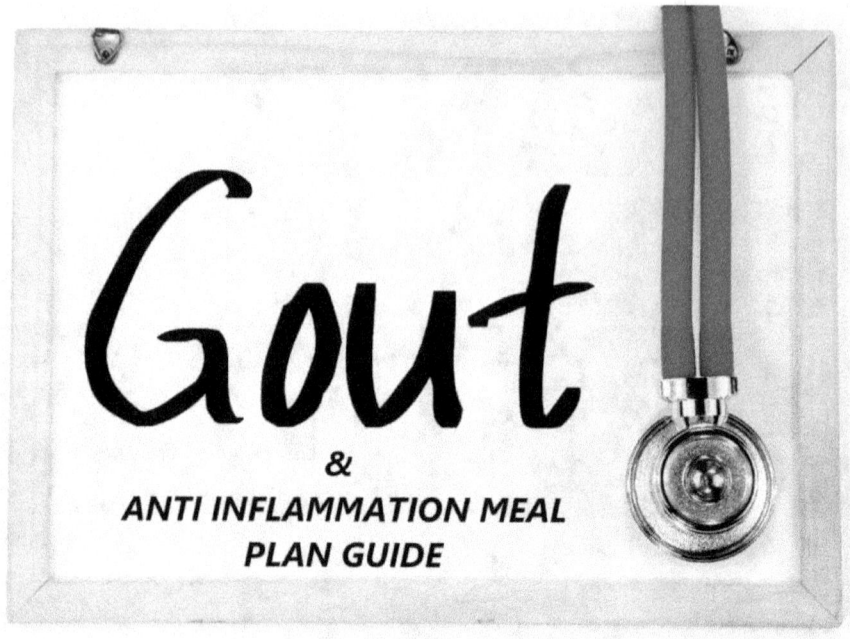

Gout

&

ANTI INFLAMMATION MEAL PLAN GUIDE

Nutritional Strategies For Reducing Inflammation Naturally

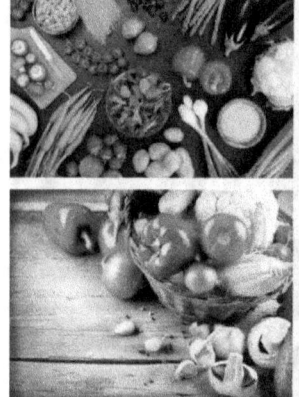

HR Research Alliance

Gout Prevention - Gout Diet - Anti Inflammatory Foods To Eat & Avoid - & More...

ANTI
INFLAMMATION

The Guide To Reducing Inflammation
JT Thorpe

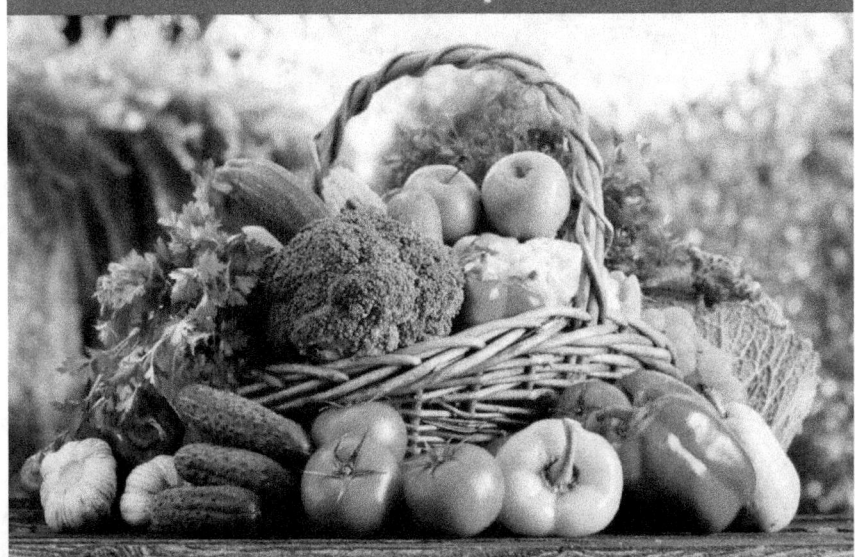

7 Day Meal Plan - Anti Inflammatory
Recipes - Lifestyle Changes - How To
Reduce Inflammation Naturally - What To
Eat - What To Avoid Eating - & Much More
Motivational & Useful Information

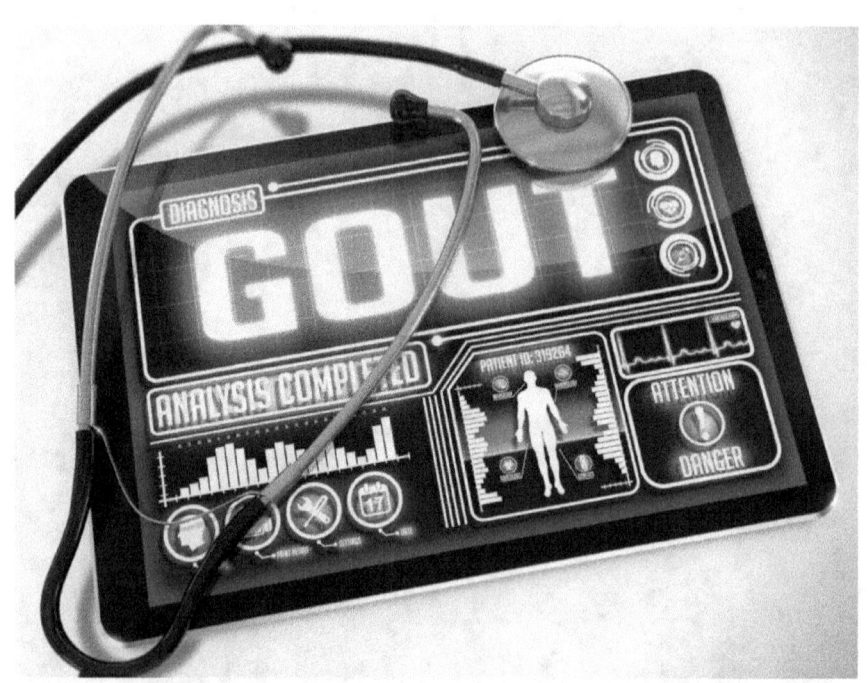

PREVENTION

A 30 Day Gout Diet & Prevention Protocol Guide Book

Gout Recipes - Lifestyle Changes - & Healthy Habits To Help Reduce Inflammation & Live Gout FREE!

Kelly Bird

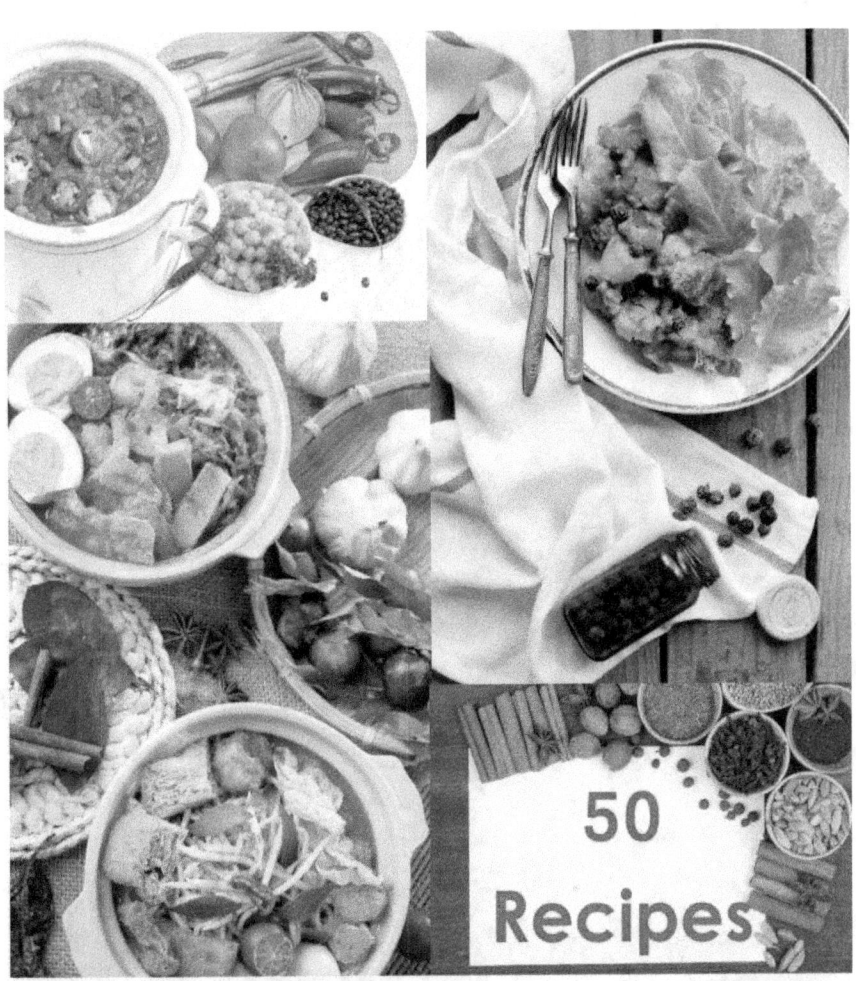

GOUT RELIEF

RECIPES

Kelly Bird

50 Recipes

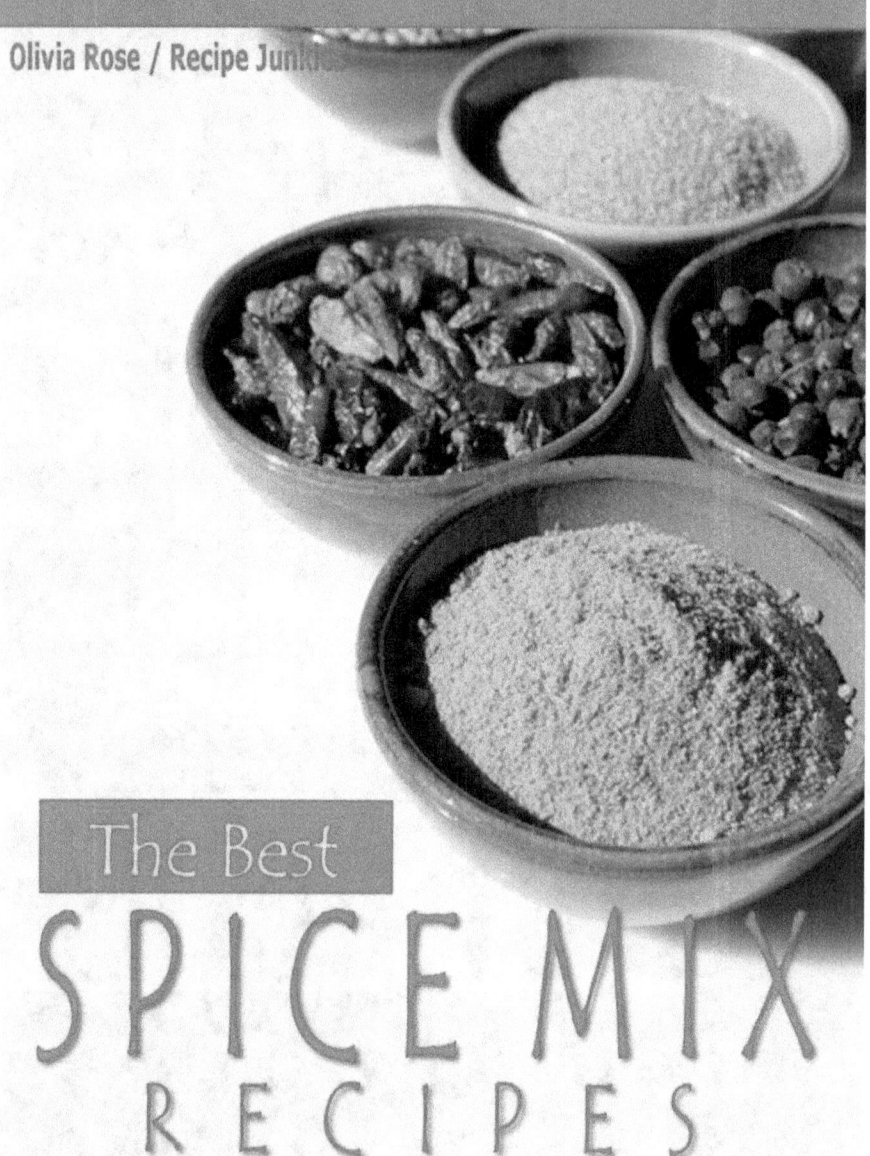

Top 50 Seasoning Recipes

Olivia Rose / Recipe Junkies

The Best

SPICE MIX

RECIPES

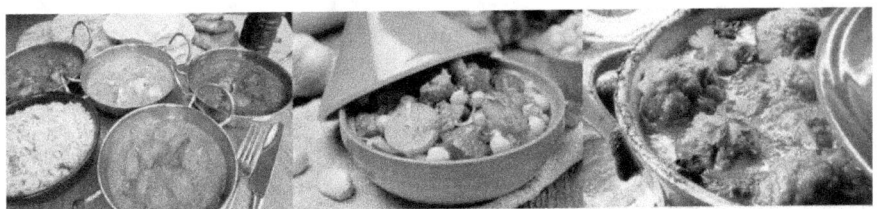

INFLAMMATION

Diet

Recipes

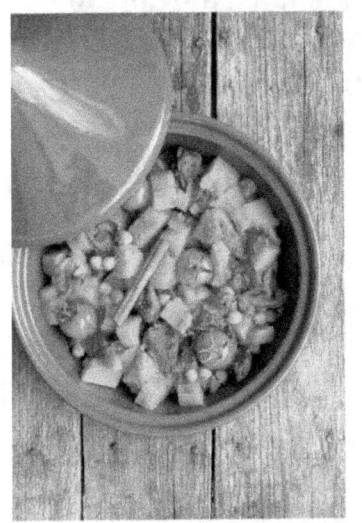

Great For Gout Relief!

70 Healthy Anti Inflammatory Crockpot & Slow Cooker Recipes

Cindy Myers

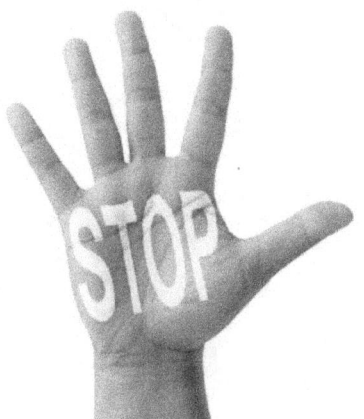

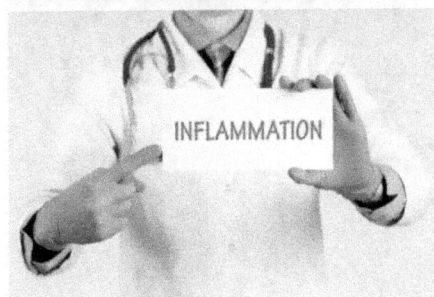

INFLAMMATION